Woman in the Bed: A Love Story

Sterling Winston Swan

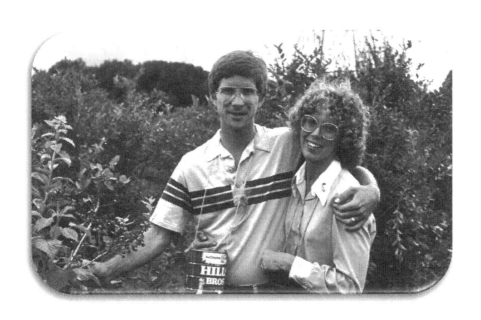

Sterling and Karen – summer 1983

For My Children

SWS Press
December 2016
Sandy, Utah
Cover Design: Allene Swan

Copyright & All Rights Reserved

Table of Contents

Introduction		9
1 ~ When God Showed Up		11
2 ~ Headaches		17
3 ~ "That Should Not Be There!"		21
4 ~ A Tumor Removed		24
5 ~ Dr. Samlowski Standing by Her Bedside		34
6 ~ Statistics in the Rear-View Mirror		41
7 ~ First Radiation		45
8 ~ Woman in the Bed		51
9 ~ "…In Sickness and in Health…"		65
10 ~ Living Life to the Fullest		75
11 ~ HCH Wellness Center		80
12 ~ It's All About Relationships		84
13 ~ The NED-in-Brain Years		90
14 ~ Personality Changes		97
15 ~ Children and God		102
16 ~ Caring For Me		107
17 ~ Clinical Trials		113

18 ~	A New Oncologist	123
19 ~	Melanoma On the March	129
20 ~	Good News, Bad News	134
21 ~	"How Did You Do That?"	137
22 ~	Perseverating	141
23 ~	"You Look Like a Million Dollars!"	151
24 ~	New Drugs	156
25 ~	Transition Months	163
26 ~	The Seizure	170
27 ~	Thanksgiving 2013	177
28 ~	Early December	187
29 ~	Christmas 2013	195
30 ~	"Candor is What We Want"	203
31 ~	The Choice	211
32 ~	Making a Family Memory	217
33 ~	Hospice	233
34 ~	Decline – Part 1	241
35 ~	Decline – Part 2	251
36 ~	End in Sight	255
37 ~	Her Soul Departs	266

38 ~ A Week of Preparations		269
39 ~ "Karen Will Always be in My Heart"		276
40 ~ Scattering Her Ashes		281
41 ~ Life After Death…		289
Appendix		295
Extend Her Legacy		297
About the Author		297

Introduction

This is a love story...

About a killer, a brave woman, her husband, four children, and dozens of other people, whose lives were touched in one way or another during a journey from life, to death, and beyond.

The killer was Stage IV melanoma cancer. Just the word "cancer" can create feelings of dread. This book is not really about those malfunctioning cells which, rather than dying, grow uncontrollably at an alarming rate and overwhelm the body's immune system. The focus here is on an incredibly courageous woman, who loved life and threw herself into the battle for her life, with a determination that stunned even experienced cancer workers.

I tell the story, a husband who became my wife's full-time caregiver and advocate. To my great surprise, in the process I experienced a changed life, an epiphany of sorts that brought me in a fresh way back to the Creator of all.

Her life was taken; many others were transformed. It is the journey of a lifetime, compressed into seven short years.

Karen Allene Swan was a beautiful woman, wife, mother, daughter, friend, and educator, with a confidence in God that extended to her last breath.

~1~

When God Showed Up

Tuesday, March 11, 2014

Karen Allene Swan, 56, died this morning, at 9:30 a.m., in her home, in the twin-size hospital bed set up in the master bedroom, surrounded by her family and a hospice nurse. In the midst of this tragedy, God showed up in a dramatic way, even as her lungs filled with fluid, causing her to struggle for every breath. She ultimately surrendered, and with a sigh, ended a courageous 7 ½ year battle with Stage IV melanoma cancer, a horrific disease that had spread to her brain, ultimately, killing her body.

Yet today, Karen's soul still lives. There is no doubt in my mind about this. None. This chapter begins to explain why.

Karen's final hours began the night before, when Camille, the hospice nurse, instructed me to give morphine to Karen every two hours via the feeding tube that snaked its way up through her right nostril, down into the small intestines. Karen had a seizure four months earlier, a seminal event that had pinched the nerve in her brain controlling her tongue, so although she could no longer swallow food, or speak without great effort, she could hear and respond by small hand motions. Hospice is all about patient comfort in the days before their likely death, and morphine has a rare ability to bring comfort to a person in the midst of their body's decline.

"Sterling," said Camille, "I am on-call tonight. If Karen has some needs that you cannot handle, rather than you calling the general nurse answering service number, then they call me, you just text me, and I will respond. I live only five minutes away and will keep my phone by my bed." Then she left.

As the sun set, family members and I moved Karen from the living room into our master bedroom, into her hospital-type bed that inclined to help her breathe. Often multiple family members were with her in the room, sitting around her, touching her, caressing her hair or holding her hands as she dozed.

By 8 p.m., she was sound asleep. As the rest of my family headed off to their rooms to relax, I gave Karen a dose of morphine, set the alarm clock for 10 p.m., then climbed into the bed next to her, the one we had slept in together for decades.

10 p.m., midnight, 2 a.m.: the alarms got me up to give Karen her dose of morphine.

3 a.m.: I awoke to Karen moving restlessly in her inclined bed, hunched over, at times breathing very sluggishly, gasping for breath. The dose of morphine I had given her an hour ago was not working. The harsh reality was, because of the aspirated fluid in her lungs, she was drowning, and the process was accelerating.

I had used all my treatment bullets. Deeply concerned, I ran downstairs to wake up Amber and Allene, my twin daughters, woke up my mother-in-law, and then texted Camille.

"Karen is in great discomfort, struggling to breathe, and the morphine is no longer working," I said.

Almost immediately, Camille texted back, "Would you like me to come?"

"Yes!"

By then, my daughters were in the master bedroom, caressing and comforting their mom. My mother-in-law soon joined us. One son, Neil, was at college thirty minutes away; one of my daughters called him and he immediately left his dorm for the house, speeding to get there, believing every minute counted. Someone in the family reached Ryan, my other son living outside Anchorage, Alaska, by phone; he soon joined us using Skype, via a laptop computer perched on a stool right next to Karen's bed.

3:30 a.m.: Camille arrived, Neil right behind her. An experienced nurse, she quickly assessed the situation and gave Karen more morphine and a decongestant, all via the feeding tube. Fortunately, the increased morphine relaxed Karen and she fell back asleep. Family members in the room, gathered around her, also feel asleep, each where they were at – chairs, master bed, and floor. Camille remained with us.

6:30 a.m.: It was lightly snowing outside. Karen awoke again, struggling. Hunching over, she was grasping for breath, heaving deeply. One of my daughters rubbed her back. I could hear liquid in her lungs. Our family cat knew something was amiss and would hardly move, curled in a tight round ball at the foot of Karen's bed.

Camille quickly prepared another strong dose of morphine and decongestant, giving it to Karen through the tube. Instinct might have had us call 911. Not with hospice. The goal was different: comfort only.

Karen was clearly dying, but we were not alone. Something supernatural was about to happen.

*****

An Appearance In Three Parts:

Part 1
7 a.m.: I walked out into the kitchen and texted Jeff Nellermoe, senior pastor of a local church, and his wife Mim. "Please pray for Karen. She is struggling; her lungs are filling with fluid, causing discomfort and difficulty breathing. A hospice nurse is here, along with my children and mother-in-law."

He was the only one I texted.

Almost immediately, Jeff texted back, "We are praying. We are house sitting only a few minutes away. Would you like us to come over?"

House sitting? Jeff had tendered his resignation just three months before this morning. He and Mim had sold 99% of their possessions and were in the process of moving to Asia to work with rural poor. The house they were in the morning of March 11 just "happened" to be literally down the hill from my home.

Fatigued and emotionally spent, I texted Jeff back, "Let me check with my children to see if they want anyone else in the house."

I never checked. My children, all adults, were too distraught experiencing their mother's rapid decline for me to even consider asking. I was just going through the motions that morning, on autopilot as it were, doing my duty and, on hindsight, receiving strength from God alone, so I never even got back to Jeff. Things were just too intense.

I went back into the bedroom, where my children were surrounding Karen – sitting by her, laying on the master bed next to her – caressing and touching her, telling her they loved her. Crying. Grieving. Karen's gasps for air had transitioned to a regular, deep sighing as though she had just run a sprint. I sat next to her, holding her hand, occasionally kissing her face.

She was clearly conscious, but no longer communicating with her hands as she had in days past. I looked carefully at her face: Her eyes stared straight ahead like she was both pulling inside herself, and looking beyond the room, somewhere else.

Part 2

7:15 a.m.: I received another text from Jeff Nellermoe. "We are sitting in our truck outside your home, praying for your family. Would you like us to come in?"

I read the text but never responded. I was too overwhelmed.

Now Jeff picks up the story:

Even though Sterling had not invited us to come over, we felt prompted to drive the five minutes to the Swan's home. I parked our old Ford truck rather haphazardly on the street, as it was early, lightly snowing, and no one was around. Sitting there, we prayed.

A few minutes passed, and as I had not received a response from Sterling to my most recent text, Mim said, "Well, I need to get to work (she was a physical education teacher at the Lutheran elementary school down the hill). Just take me to work and you can come back if you want."

I started the truck's engine, but rather than pull straight ahead and take Mim to work, I backed up, parked legally against the curb, and turned it off.

Mim looked at me and said, "What are you doing? I need to get to work."

"Mim," I said, "just as I started the truck engine to take you to work, I heard an audible female voice clearly tell me to go inside that house."

"You heard WHAT," said Mim?

" I heard a woman tell me to go inside that house, and we are going in."

So we did.

Part 3

Now the story returns to me:

Next thing I know, my daughter, Allene, said, "Hey, dad, Jeff and Mim are in the house." I walked out to the living room to greet them, explained that Karen has aspirated fluid into her lungs, and was slowly drowning.

We exchanged hugs. They asked if they could come in and give her a blessing. I impulsively said, "Yes."

I brought them into the master bedroom, where they quietly and compassionately greeted everyone. Walking over to Karen's bed, Jeff and Mim knelt right beside her, their faces even with hers. I don't know how acute Karen's senses were at this point, but I sure hope she could hear what Jeff and Mim did next.

Jeff took out his iPhone, found some comforting verses from the Bible (including Psalm 23), then read them out loud. Next, he took out a small vial of oil and anointed Karen's forehead, a ritual drawing from rich Biblical and historical tradition. After this, he and Mim sang a couple short songs. Finally, Jeff prayed.

Their mission complete, they got up, hugged Karen and the other family members, and left.

Two hours later, at 9:30 a.m., Karen died.

*****

A week later, shortly after Karen's memorial, I met Jeff at Starbucks and asked him if he had any idea whose voice that was, the one that clearly told him to go into my home. "Not Mim's, that's for sure. Karen's? An angel? I don't know. But, the voice was female and crystal clear."

I asked, "How many times have something like this happened in your 21 years of working in a church?"

"Only four," said Jeff, a highly educated man not prone to emotional excesses or making things up for effect. On the other hand, he is very tuned into what God is doing in this world, and on the morning of March 11, 2014, he and Mim were clearly brought to my home, summoned really.

Their timely appearance, impossible for me to script even in the best of circumstances, was as though someone had pulled back the curtain shielding my human eyes from the Heavenly realm, just enough so I could see an involved Creator – certainly not someone who heals every one – but who cares in the midst of hardship, grief, and loss.

Jeff and Mim were also profoundly changed by the experience that morning. Alas, their story will wait for another telling.

*****

My wife died that morning. With one last, long, deep breath, Karen Allene Swan was gone, in an instant seeing her Savior, Jesus Christ, face to face. She left her family, all she loved.

Watching someone I loved, more than life itself, die, is simply a horrific experience, like someone had just kicked me in the stomach. I miss Karen profoundly. She was the light of my life.

Were that the end of the story – of a person returning to dust – I doubt I would be writing this book. Her death did not have the final word, her ashes merely the ultimate fate of us all.

Far from it.

On that wintry, sorrowful morning, a seed of hope was planted in my life. That hope not only sustained me after she died but also gave me understanding of how God had walked beside Karen, my family and I, during the long years we battled cancer together.

That journey also began in my home, in October 2006.

~2~

Headaches

Headaches!

Karen, 49, started getting them regularly around mid-September 2006.

Historically, I was the one that typically got headaches, mainly stress-related. Karen, not so much. She was a strong Dutch woman – mother, a part-time educator in a community school cooperative, physically active – so this pain was a caution flag.

Menopause? Perhaps. Sinus pressure? Ear infection? We started running down the list of possibilities based on life experience. What we did not consider was cancer. Who would? Just the word itself quickly leads to thoughts about suffering, twisted bodies, pain, and mortality.

Initially, Karen tried to manage the pain with over-the-counter pain relievers and laying on our bed at just the right angle. That worked, but only for so long. It got to the point where she could barely drag herself out of bed, much less head off to teach, only to come back home and collapse on the bed, trying to find the increasingly elusive, comfortable position.

September drifted into October, the pain escalating upwards nearly every day.

Monday morning, October 16: Karen could no longer cope. Deeply concerned and baffled, I held her arm as we walked together to the car, off to a hastily arranged appointment with a family practice physician recommended by a friend. Karen was in such good health that, at this point, she did not even have her own general practice doctor.

We got to the clinic early so that Karen could have a blood draw, providing critical information for the upcoming evaluation. Eventually the physician entered the room and, after a few pleasantries, began asking the typical diagnostic questions:
- Why are you here?
- How long have you had these symptoms?

- Are you on any medications?
- Do you drink alcohol?
- Have you had any falls or concussions?

Next, the physician had Karen lay down on the exam table, where she performed an exam around the abdominal area. At one point, the doctor asked Karen to turn onto her right side. As Karen did, she let out a loud cry of pain. It startled me, as Karen has a very high pain threshold. Clearly, something was wrong.

What?

With that painful cry, the physical exam portion of the appointment ended.

"You can get up now," remarked the physician.

Karen could not get up. The pain had immobilized her, so I went over and helped lift her to a sitting position, easing her off the exam table, and finally over to a chair. As she sat next to me, resting against my shoulder, I watched the physician staring intently at the blood work data on the exam room's computer monitor, as if to say, "Speak to me, numbers. Tell me what is wrong."

She scrolled through the pages, pausing, waiting for insight. Karen's blood pressure and other vital signs were normal. There were no clues there.

Finally, the doctor turned to us and said that she was not able to determine the cause of Karen's pain, and recommended that I take Karen directly to one of the larger hospitals in the Valley for evaluation, as they would have more resources to diagnosis the problem.

*****

Arm-in-arm, I slowly walked Karen out to the car, helped her climb into the passenger seat, and then off we went, to a hospital about twenty minutes away. Large and relatively close to our home, this would allow me to get Karen evaluated and pick Neil, age 13, up from school mid-afternoon. It all made perfect sense, except that our world was about to cave in.

When Karen and I walked into the ER, to our shock, the place was undergoing a remodel. Staff told me the wait would be about an hour; I decided to stay there, rather than drive another 20 minutes to the University of Utah hospital, further north, further away from our home and Neil's school. I got Karen settled into the rather small, noisy waiting room – with traumas, children, dueling T.V.s, and constant, intense hustle and bustle – and then began filling out the reams of paperwork covering insurance, medical history, symptoms, permission to treat, etc.

Unfortunately, Karen was in for a wait, and ER waiting rooms are not calming, comfortable places, but rather loud, chaotic, mixing bowls of hurting people and their loved ones with all sorts of traumas and issues. I elected to leave Karen there, alone, so that I could run to Neil's school, pick him up and bring him home. Once I had him settled at home, I headed back to the hospital ER.

Why didn't I have a friend pick him up? It really didn't occur to me, since I was still thinking that this was a "one-off" problem with Karen's pain, so that, of course, we would be home once the ER doc saw her and gave her meds for the pain. Who in normal life anticipates something more serious? No one.

By the time I made that long driving loop, ninety minutes had elapsed. As I walked into the ER waiting room, there Karen was, now sitting on the floor, searching for a way, any way, to lessen some of the pain in her head. I promptly headed to the ER check-in desk to find out what in the world was going on.

Apologetic, staff advised an additional wait. Disgusted, I called the University of Utah Hospital's ER number and ask about their wait time: 45 minutes. Apparently it was a busy Monday afternoon all over the Valley.

After a quick calculation, I decided we would stay at the present hospital because of proximity to home, without knowing that six hours later, Karen would be transported to the University Hospital via ambulance. At the end of the day, proximity to home would be the least of my concerns.

"Hospital time" is typically slower than normal time. Things just take longer, for a wide variety of reasons. So it went that Monday afternoon. Fatigue and frustration were starting to set in with Karen and me, to the point where I shifted gears, with one foot out of the ER Waiting Room to get the car and take Karen to the University Hospital just as staff called her name.

"Karen Swan!!"

They led us to a small exam room sandwiched behind bare drywall and plastic sheets hiding the construction. A medical assistant (MA) asked what brought us in. Karen haltingly explained the pain in her skull, and I gave a short synopsis of the earlier visit to the family practice physician. I asked when we would see the physician; it would be soon, just as soon as the MA took Karen's vitals and "consulted" with the physician.

Soon, the ER physician appeared; one question followed another. Much like our previous physician experience earlier in the day, this doctor could not determine the symptoms' cause through her line of questioning, so she ordered a computed tomography (CT) scan of Karen's brain.

While waiting for the scan, staff inserted an IV line into one of Karen's veins so she could receive pain medication and a saline solution for hydration. Within minutes, Karen's pain began subsiding, just in time for us to enjoy the sandwiches and drinks someone had ordered. Nicely done.

More staff appeared, whisking Karen off for a CT, only to bring her back in less than a half hour. "Wow," I thought to myself, "that was fast." Her pain, now completely under control, allowed us to finally talk calmly for the first time all day. Words spilled out rapid fire. We were in a fog. Baffled. I assured her that Neil was fine, safe at home, eating dinner and studying.

While Karen is one tough woman, this afternoon, she was numb. Exhausted. Afraid. All these years, she had brought our children to see doctors when problems arose. Now, she was the patient, awaiting the scan results.

~3~

"That Should Not Be There!"

This particular hospital's scans were still in the pre-digital era, which meant that when the ER physician came back, she carried a 15x20 inch manila envelope containing the CT images. "I have already looked at these images and consulted with a radiologist. Let me show you," she said as she inserted one of the large film negatives into a wall-mounted viewer-reader so common in hospital exam rooms back then.

On went the display's backlight, and strikingly, there was the outline of Karen's entire brain. True to what appears in popular culture, most of the brain image was in shades of darker gray.

Most.

The physician pointed to a lighter gray, milky-colored orb, about the size of a tangerine, on the right side of Karen's brain, just above her ear, and said, "That should not be there!"

In an instant, those five words changed my family forever.

"This orb likely indicates a tumor," said the physician. "Because this hospital does not have the expertise to deal with complex brain issues, I recommend that we immediately transfer you to the University of Utah hospital. We will start the transfer process just as soon as you give the word. Please discuss this and let the staff know your decision."

With that, the physician and staff left Karen and me alone to talk. Karen was a practical, no-nonsense person. She had a zest for life that would not stop, so the decision was clear. "I want to go to the University Hospital," she said. "I want to fight this, get this thing out of my head."

I walked out into the hallway, flagged down a nurse and told her we wanted to go to the University Hospital. With this green light, the administrative wheels to make the transfer happen started turning.

There are several very large hospitals just in the Salt Lake Valley, all of which regularly deal with complex brain issues. On hindsight, there is no question in my mind that the ER physician's University Hospital recommendation initiated one of many, many divine events that would guide Karen's life over the next seven years. Why? In just a few days, Karen would be recovering from brain surgery, in a comfortable room at the Huntsman Cancer Hospital, a place that would become her second home and where she would find hope and healing.

*****

Next step was to get Karen to our car so I could drive her to the University Hospital, right? No. The physician popped into the exam room again, only to say that she strongly recommended transport via ambulance in the event Karen had a seizure.

Seizure?

Ambulance?

Is it that serious? My world, of kids with ear infections, tonsillectomies, and E. coli poisoning, suddenly got a lot more complex. Picking my battles, I agreed to the ambulance, but in the back of my mind I was also thinking money. That ambulance ride was going to be expensive. While a reasonable consideration, in the big scheme of things, this cost concern was really quite absurd. Over the next 7½ years, I would have enough medical bills and insurance explanation-of-benefits (EOBs) to wallpaper my house, and in light of medical charges coming just over the horizon, an ambulance bill was pocket change.

Karen's decision set in motion a carefully choreographed drama, including staff that would cycle in and out of our exam room in rapid-fire succession: RNs, MAs, billing specialists, the ER physician, and even a person bringing more sandwiches.

In between all these faces, Karen and I were alone, to face our own shock, tears, and utter disbelief.

Neil?

Oh, what about Neil at home? I picked up the exam room phone and dialed the Binghams, a family that lived across the street from us in Sandy. Jamie – wife, mother, and faithful friend – answered. I blurted out a couple of words, only to hang up, crying.

Jamie told me later that night that she had used her caller ID to try calling back, but only got as far as the hospital's switchboard.

Because of privacy laws, it was a dead-end from there. She was unable to track me down.

A few minutes later, I grabbed Karen's cell phone, walked outside the hospital, and called Jamie again. I told her that Karen likely had a brain tumor, we were at St. Marks going to the U, and could she go over and sit with Neil?

Of course, she would. Our many neighbors were there for us for over seven years.

As I walked back into the exam room, the ambulance team did, too, rolling a gurney. Like the professionals they were, they carefully lifted her off the hospital bed, over to the gurney, strapped her in and off they went, weaving down the halls out to the ambulance.

"That was fast," I thought as I ran to my car. "I am going to follow the ambulance."

Not.

It was long gone.

"How do I get to the U of U hospital?"

"Where is the ER?"

"Who is going to care for my wife?"

I wove my way through Salt Lake City, up to the University area, finally arriving at the hospital, one of the State's flagship Trauma Center facilities, a huge building bathed in light against a dark fall sky.

~4~

A Tumor Removed

"Where is Karen," I thought as I walked from the parking structure to the hospital's ER entrance? "Did I get here before her?"

No, the ambulance had arrived and she was already in an ER exam room. When I joined her there, an ER physician was going through the standard Q&A assessment process. We had heard those same questions earlier in the day. Twice.

I was learning another lesson: I was now a caregiver. What did that mean? There was no roadmap, no class I had taken, and no script to follow, just some vows said long ago, "…in sickness and in health." Caregiving is a shifting dynamic between husband and wife, child and aging parent, friend to friend. As a wife and mother, Karen not only took care of her own medical needs, but those of our children, and often, mine. Now, the roles would change; in many ways, caregiving became a full-time job for me.

Even on Day 1 of our journey, I decided to jump into the caring role by advocating for Karen in this ER room, by providing the physician with a complete chronological history going back several weeks, an overview which he told me he appreciated. I remember him carefully listening to me, occasionally looking over to Karen for cues that I was accurately speaking for her, and then we would continue. Over the next seven years, she and I found that this tag-team arrangement worked very well, resulting in our establishing strong relationships with her physicians and the dozens of support staff. They obtained the all-important status information, and we built trust with her medical team, that we were engaged and "owned" Karen's care.

Karen was exhausted. When I explained to the physician that she had been up all day and had not received pain medication for some time, he ordered more. Then, I showed him the film of the CT taken of Karen's brain. With that data alone, he recommended a Magnetic Resonance Image (MRI) scan, which would produce an image of greater clarity, and since the University Hospital was completely digital, this image could easily be shared with other medical staff. Finally, since the CT scan alone indicated some sort of tumor, he recommended Karen's formal admission to the hospital, a first for her.

Once "hospital time" worked its mysterious ways, Karen was officially admitted. Staff wheeled her to a private in-patient room, up several floors in the main hospital building. In this complex web of care, the next person who appeared was a nurse, explaining the details of the night ahead. We learned that along with regular checks of her vitals and IV line, she would receive physician-prescribed pain meds every four hours, and yes, plenty of food. In the morning, a neurosurgeon would swing by Karen's room to discuss her situation.

Until that happened, Karen should get some sleep. So should I.

Could I stay with her overnight? Yes, the chair I was in did recline (like a Lay-Z-Boy), but the hospital's older design meant that there was no real bed for me. The nurse recommended that since I lived relatively close, I go home, sleep in my own bed, and then come back early tomorrow morning when Karen would be awake. "She will be well cared for," was the nurse's reassuring comment.

I decided to go home.

As I drove those thirty minutes, I made brief calls to my three older children, all attending Biola University that fall in La Mirada, California. The news shocked them. We agreed to talk more the next day.

By then I was home. Jamie, the neighbor who was watching Neil, greeted me as I opened the front door. It was 10 p.m. She had been dozing on the couch; Neil was as in bed. I gave Jamie a summary of what was going on, she gave me a much-appreciated hug, I walked her home, and then I got ready for bed myself.

I remember lying in that king-size bed, the one that Karen and I had shared for many years, trying to wrap my mind around the fact that she was now in a hospital room thirty minutes away, facing a crisis of unknown proportions. My thoughts and emotions were jumbled and disoriented. I have never felt so alone, to the point where I broke down crying. I called a good friend, stumbled through a brief explanation, and asked him to pray with me.

I was not sure if that helped or not, because when I hung up the phone, I wept again. Tears, especially early on, would become my frequent companion on this journey. Do prayers make the pain go away? Not always. Not usually. Do tears represent unbelief? Hardly.

*****

I can't remember how much I slept that night, or the nature of my dreams, only that I was up early, ate, showered, and headed back to the University Hospital. As I pulled into the hospital's parking garage, Amber called. On her lips was the key question: What does the tumor in the brain mean?

"I don't know," I replied. "I will call you as soon as we meet with a doctor." With that, I walked up to Karen's room.

Karen had slept well. Thanks, morphine! She was eating breakfast as I walked in, so we started voicing facts, feelings, our children, and unknown of what is next. We had no idea what we were in for. Perhaps that was good. There was a tumor in her brain; we knew that much. What was it? How to get it out? It was too early in the game to think cancer, much less a life-threatening disease.

Soon after I arrived, a nurse came in, asked how Karen was feeling (using a 1 to 10 point scale: 1 terrible, 10 great), and told us that one of the hospital's neurosurgeons would come in later that morning to discuss what they had learned from the MRI performed last night and another one done earlier in the morning before I arrived. "You will like Dr. Jensen," I remember her saying. "The patients and staff think he is one of the best." While we waited, I made some calls – to Karen's folks, close friends, and members of our church – explaining the situation and asking for prayer.

Dr. Randy Jensen, a neurosurgeon, arrived nearly to the minute after I had finished my last phone call and chased down a cup of coffee. A very personable, middle-aged man, with a disarming smile and an appreciation of my humor, Dr. Jensen grabbed a chair, introduced himself, and asked Karen a bit more of her history. Then, he launched into a discussion about her recent MRI images, painting a picture that involved a whole new vocabulary with very serious implications.

Dr. Jensen is a brilliant, experienced, well-respected neurosurgeon, and at the same time, a very kind, compassionate, humble human being, a rather rare combination for someone so high up the medical food chain. We would grow to trust him with Karen's brain, in ways that we have never trusted a physician before. In just twenty-four hours, I was twice reminded that Karen and I were not alone. Someone was aware of our needs. We were led to the University Hospital for her care, and Dr. Jensen would be her neurosurgeon, helping to preserve her life for many years to come.

Dr. Jensen explained that the tumor, above the right ear, in the right temporal lobe of Karen's brain, was type unknown. It was essentially spherical, about the size of a tangerine. Spherical was good, in contrast to other types of tumors, which have fingers that squeeze their way through nooks and crannies of a person's brain. He laid out treatment options: surgery, radiation, drugs, and/or nothing. Each option had trade-offs; he explained those, too. Karen and I wanted to know. Information was power.

Based on Karen's overall physical health, strong personality, the spherical nature of the tumor, and later treatment of the area with targeted radiation, Dr. Jensen recommended surgery (resection) to remove as much of the tumor as possible.

"Will I face impairment by the removal of that tumor and some functioning brain tissue," Karen asked? "Be straight with me."

Dr. Jensen made clear that brain surgery is no small matter, as brain damage, or even death from infection, is always a possibility. In Karen's case, he believed the likelihood of a positive outcome was good. As for impairment, while the temporal lobes are thought to have a major role in processing and storing visual, language and emotional data, the two lobes – one on the right, the other, left – seem to support one another, perhaps redundantly. In theory, damage one, and the other can take up the slack.

At least as of the fall of 2006, science was only beginning to understand the role of the various brain lobes and how they worked together. With a sly smile, he said that the right temporal lobe is "like a spare tire. We aren't completely sure what it does, or how removing it will affect your person."

Although it was dark humor, the "spare tire" comment would come to characterize much of Karen's cancer journey; there would be lots and lots of educated judgments, not certainties. By engaging with the physicians, and allowing for ambiguities, yes, even dark humor, we actually arrived at better outcomes than if we had expected omniscient surgeons and oncologists.

We learned that while tumors typically compress brain tissue, that tissue will normally spring back, filling part or the entire cavity left from the tumor's removal. In addition, surgery on this type of spherical tumor can remove about 70% of the malignant tissue, radiation can kill another 20%, but unfortunately, tumor cells remain. It's just the nature of the beast. That's where chemotherapy, or something more advanced, comes in, that is, if a patient can tolerate the side effects of the medicines.

Which path would Karen choose? Without hesitation, she said, "I want the surgery. How soon can it happen? Get that tumor out of my brain."

Dr. Jensen pulled out his smart phone, made a couple of entries, found that he had an open slot on Thursday, two days hence, and added Karen's name to the roster. His final comment: Over the next 24 hours, various hospital staff would come to our room and explain the surgery process in detail.

*****

The decision made, Dr. Jensen departed. There sat Karen and I, looking at each other as bewilderment, uncertainty, resignation, shock, and hope washed up on us like waves of the sea. Yet, we had spent our lives under the conviction that God is not "out there," but here, present with us, even as our little boat pushed further down into a canyon filled with dark, turbulent waters. Can confusion, fear, and faith exist side by side? On that morning, in us, they did.

I had one urgent phone call to make, to at least one my three oldest children, explaining that their mother was scheduled for brain surgery this Thursday. Please come. Tell the others.

I spent the rest of the morning and early afternoon with Karen, talking details, the shock of it all, and gathering information from the stream of hospital staff that started to appear, all with the purpose of coordinating the upcoming surgery. Before I left the hospital, I also made one other call, to Blue Cross/Blue Shield, my medical insurance company.

"Here is the situation," I said to the person in their call center. "Explain to me how this all works. Is there prior approval necessary? What is covered? How does the hospital communicate with you on billing issues?" After that, I left to pick up Neil from school and head home.

After I explained some general details to Neil, 13, I made dinner for the two of us, and then said goodbye. A family friend volunteered to let him stay at their home. I went back to the hospital. Karen had rested well throughout the afternoon. She had just finished dinner. We talked more, prayed some, and soon, it was time for sleep, for us both. She drifted off and I headed home, soon to return.

*****

Wednesday morning.

One of my three older children called to say they were on their way. It was a 720-mile drive; if all went well, we would see them early evening. I scurried around the house getting beds ready, and then left for the hospital.

Come early evening, the emotional intensity level jumped a couple notches as my three older children arrived at the hospital. They were understandably tired from the long drive, yet deeply concerned about their mother. Neil also showed up, brought by a family friend. The five of us grabbed spots in that small room, bantering back and forth with Karen and each other, trying to make sense of events so far and what was to come.

What was to come? Years ago, one of my daughters, then only age two, had surgery to reopen a portion of her skull that had prematurely closed. A pediatric neurosurgeon had performed the procedure, but it was skeletal, not inside the brain itself. Karen's surgery was qualitatively different, and as I explained the details to my children, all any of us could do was hope, and shower Karen with love. Which we did! We were in the midst of humbling reality: we did not know what we did not know. Time would fill in many of those gaps. There were no guarantees.

It was soon time for the five of us to leave so that everyone could get some sleep. We headed to the Sandy home, where my children had all grown up; now they had returned, to support their mother in the fight of her life.

*****

Thursday: Surgery day.

Back to Karen's room we went, only to find her moved to a surgery preparation area. Staff guided us over to the new area, another small, private room, now filled with the family and an ever-changing assortment of medical staff. It was a time of waiting, of nervous laughter, touching, and coffee. This brain surgery was a major production, no question about it.

Nursing staff regularly came in and out, checking vitals, keeping us updated. The anesthesiologist and his two residents popped in, explained the procedures he would use to fully sedate Karen, and when the surgery was over, bring her back to consciousness. We asked questions, he answered, and as they left, Dr. Jensen came in for a last minute update.

I was glad that my four children could hear all the medical details directly from the physicians. On one hand, it is very sobering; however, good information can help counter fear and rumor.

Now, things were moving at a rapid clip. More support staff appeared, unplugging cords, releasing bed wheel brakes, pushing her out of the prep room and into the wide hospital corridors. The five of us walked beside the bed, alternately holding her hands, tossing out light humor, and quietly pondering the implications of this day.

Finally, we were there, the surgery transition area just outside a surgery suite. This was as far as we could go. It was time for hugs, kisses, and well wishes.

Then…she was gone.

Whisked away for surgery.

It was surreal.

None of us had ever experienced anything like this before. There was a possibility we would never see our wife and mother again, or that she would survive the surgery, but with neurological or bacterial complications. I did not think about these possibilities. This is what I allowed: Karen was going in for surgery, Dr. Jensen was competent, and the resection would take some time. All we could do was wait, pray, hope, worry, and call people all across the country to stand with us.

*****

Oh, yes, that's right, we needed breakfast! Although the hospital had a decent cafeteria, the staff recommended we take a short hike, just up the hill, to the Huntsman Cancer Hospital's Pointe restaurant on the hospital's sixth floor. Apparently it was higher quality, reasonably priced food, freshly cooked by chefs, and came with a sweeping view of the Salt Lake valley. So while Ryan ran Neil to school, my daughters and I took a walk. All the hype proved true, and then some. The Huntsman Hospital and Pointe restaurant were beautifully designed, warm, calming places.

After breakfast, we were in for a long wait in the hospital's surgery waiting area, as total expected surgery time was four hours. Close to that time estimate, waiting area staff notified me that Karen was out of surgery and that Dr. Jensen would soon join us for an update.

They were right. He appeared, still in his Scrubs, waiving us over to an adjoining patient consulting room for greater privacy.

"The resection of the tumor was a success," he said. "There were no complications. The spherical nature of the tumor made removal easier than other forms of tumors. Karen is in recovery, coming out of deep anesthesia. When she is able to have family come to her, staff will come get you. She will be in recovery for an hour or so, then moved to another area for close monitoring. Tissue from the tumor will undergo full biopsy overnight, and while we should know by tomorrow the exact nature of the cells, rapid pathology results performed at the time of surgery indicate it is melanoma cancer.

"One of my colleagues, an oncologist, will visit Karen tomorrow morning with more information on the pathology results. Sterling, I recommend you attend."

Dr. Jensen invited questions. We had none. It was enough that the surgery was a success.

Eventually, we joined Karen in the recovery area. She was groggy, yet managed a small smile, part of her nature. We smothered her with hugs. A nurse explained that Karen would remain in recovery for a bit longer, and then staff would move her to a surgery recovery room. I could stay with her in the recovery area.

With that, my children left for home.

Karen rebounded quickly, which meant she was promptly moved to a surgery recovery area with a low patient-to-nurse ratio.

Surgery, I would learn, is emotionally and physically exhausting for the patient, so more than anything, Karen needed sleep, lots of it. Once staff got her settled in her recovery room, as forecast, she quickly fell asleep. I extended the room's recliner chair and tried to do the same.

"Oh, right, I need food. Time for dinner." I left my cell number with Karen's nurse and went hunting for the hospital's cafeteria.

Brain surgery is intense science and skill, on an organ that controls everything about a person. Put stress on that organ, remove part of it, radiate it, introduce drugs into it, and there are often side effects, unique for each person. When I arrived back from dinner, Karen was awake, complaining that she could hear every little sound in the adjoining nurses' work area. Beeping sounds emitted by the IV and blood pressure machines exacerbated this noise sensitivity. She noticed every little ray of light coming through the window shades and the door blinds, even though both were fully drawn and the room lights off. Surgery had somehow heightened her sensual awareness.

Nursing staff, made aware of Karen's sound sensitively, tried to muffle their conversations as much as possible. In addition, I did my best to darken the room even more. In an attempt at levity, I joked that she could probably hear an ant crawling across the floor.

Oops – not funny.

Note to self: don't try that again.

I was exhausted. After making sure Karen was comfortable, I gave up on the recliner, told the nurses I was going home, and left. "Hospital staff are all around, keeping an eye on her. She needs to sleep. I need to sleep. I am going home," were my thoughts. This all made rational sense.

Karen told me some days later that she had slept fitfully that night, feeling terribly alone. No one she knew was there to comfort her. I felt awful about this. It was part of the caregiver's steep learning curve, not realizing just how much loneliness a patient can experience in a hospital, even with staff all around. In the future, I determined that when Karen was in-patient, I would be there, too, no matter what. I would soon discover that the Huntsman Cancer Hospital had this need, along with other caregiver creature comforts, figured out.

Although lonely, Karen received an unexpected gift that night. Looking for a distraction, she decided to channel surf the TV and landed on a local public television station. What was on? A pianist was playing a concerto, filled with powerful, expressive, beautiful sounds, on an instrument that Karen loved and played. She told me it soothed her like nothing else, a gift that chased away much of her gloom. Months later, she would study the connection between music and the brain. This was the first of many experiences with music soothing her during brain scans and radiation treatments.

~5~

Dr. Samlowski Standing By Her Bedside

I drove to the University Hospital bright and early the next morning to find Karen sitting up in bed, surprisingly alert. Nursing staff told us Dr. Jensen would drop later in the morning to check on Karen, standard procedure after any type of surgery. In the meantime, she wanted to talk, so we did, about many things.

Soon, there was a knock at the door. It was not Dr. Jensen. One of his colleagues, Dr. Wolfram Samlowski, entered the room, with a fellow close behind. Like a complex stage play, these professionals were part of a well-designed medical team that would make Karen's long battle with cancer possible.

In medical parlance, Drs. Jensen and Samlowski were "attending" physicians, highly experienced doctors who both cared for patients, and trained students, either fresh out of medical school, or years down the road in their pursuits of particular medical knowledge and careers. The three categories of students were: interns – 1st-year doctors out of medical school; residents – doctors in years 2-4 following medical school; and fellows – doctors in years 5-6 after medical school. The University's medical school meant that there were often students from at least one of these groups accompanying the attending physicians as they went about their work.

"Dr. Jensen asked me to stop by to see you this morning, as we have obtained the results of the tissue biopsy from Karen's tumor surgery."

With that, he walked to Karen's left side, explained that he was an oncologist at the Huntsman, and asked Karen how she was feeling. I carefully watched him interacting with her; I saw respect, experience, empathy, and seriousness, all wrapped around an effort to communicate important information and size up what type of person she was.

Then he delivered the news: the overnight biopsy confirmed melanoma cancer.

Cancer?

I barely knew how to spell the word. Now my wife had it?

Melanoma cancer is what brought him to Karen's room that Friday morning. He told us he had spent his entire 30-year career fighting the scourge of this dreaded, tenacious disease. It was, he said, not only his profession but also his passion, which I heard and saw very clearly in his voice tone, body language, as well as vocabulary. This passion, for his patients and possible cures, was at the core of what we would see lived out in this man for the next seven years. His intelligence, experience, personality, and drive are what made him the ideal physician to care for Karen, and why, down the road, he made himself available 24 hours a day via email. Icing on the cake: He encouraged my questions and laughed at my jokes. I liked him a lot.

It seemed that melanoma was piling on, as Dr. Samlowski added that a CT scan performed earlier in the week of Karen's torso area showed a mass in her right lung. About the size of a golf ball, this tumor was probably melanoma. A biopsy would confirm it.

How did this happen? What did it all mean? What was next? I heard the words, but on that morning at least, their meaning largely escaped me.

He explained that melanoma likes to metastasize (spread) to the brain, so removing the tumor, and then radiating the tumor cavity, were the first two steps. "Stabilize the brain," was the medical shorthand. While surgery had removed the tumor, the brain was in trauma (mostly swelling, and some bleeding) from the operation. Lots of rest at home would allow the brain to calm down and heal. Once her brain recovered, radiation would follow.

Before Karen was released from the hospital, he told us that staff would schedule her for an appointment with him in about three weeks, a 45-minute consultation, at the Huntsman Cancer Hospital, to get the lay-of-the-land on how to proceed. "Until then," he said, "you need to recover from this surgery. It is one step at a time when fighting cancer."

Finally, he explained that effective cancer treatment requires a team approach. He and Dr. Jensen, and their colleagues would work in an inter-disciplinary way to provide Karen with the best possible care.

I wanted to scream, "I insist that you remove all the bad cells immediately!" Unfortunately, this is not how the battle was going to go. It would be a long, intense, multi-year war, not a one-shot, magic treatment that would eliminate the cells that were wrecking havoc in Karen's body.

*****

Clearly, Dr. Samlowski was a Godsend. We would learn that colleagues viewed him as a trailblazer in the field, a man motivated to think outside the box because of loyalty to his patients. Dr. Jensen was the same way. Not only were they colleagues, but friends, and their advocacy for Karen was breathtaking as they worked together in ways that are impossible to describe in mere words. I saw it played out in dozens of different ways over seven years. I firmly believe those men set Karen on a path that profoundly contributed to her living way beyond the statistical average. Frankly, I seriously doubt Karen would have gone beyond those averages had she been treated somewhere else. We were in exactly the right place.

With that, our brief introduction to Dr. Samlowski was over; he and the fellow left Karen and I to start processing this bombshell news. More news was coming. Dr. Jensen came in shortly afterward (rounding, as hospital physicians call it), and concisely explained to Karen and I the outcome of her surgery. Among other things, he was quite pleased that the tumor was spherical, explaining that he had a good view of the tumor and it came out rather easily. He echoed Dr. Samlowski's words, "We stabilize the brain first, so you need to rest at home. You will see Dr. Samlowski, followed by a radiation oncologist, who will explore the radiation options with you. That's a few weeks away. For now, rest is the prescription."

Was this all a dream? Would I wake up soon? How were we to wrap our minds around this? Good thing we did not know what was coming. "One day at a time," would be our core mindset for the next seven years.

Karen was rebounding so well that staff decided to move her down one notch in the post-surgery recovery room care, from an area with a very low patient/nurse ratio (the neuro intensive care unit), to a unit with moderate nursing/patient care ratios. That meant that she would share a room with another patient. Initially, this did not seem like a big deal, but once the move occurred, and as the hours stretched on, things soured. First, she became increasingly agitated. Second, because of limited space, my children and I had a hard time hanging out in Karen's portion of the shared room at the same time. Finally, the other patient was struggling, requiring lots of nursing attention.

It was, in a word, an annoyance.

After I complained about the situation, hospital staff kicked around some possible solutions, and one bubbled to the top: move Karen to the Huntsman Cancer Hospital (HCH, or the Huntsman, for short) for the last few days of her recovery. It was a simple idea that offered comfort for my family. University Hospital staff called the Huntsman, they had space, and within an hour, she was there. Thankfully, the Huntsman Cancer Hospital was a preferred provider with my insurance, a huge financial relief to me.

The Huntsman was all about treating the whole person. They didn't just talk about that in their PR literature, they did it. That facility would be life giving for Karen. People traveled from all over the Intermountain area to receive treatment there. We lived thirty minutes away.

Her Huntsman Hospital room was large, clean, and comfortable, with plenty of chairs for family to gather, and a sweeping view of the Salt Lake Valley. Staff was incredibly competent and attentive. Patient meals were of highest quality, and the restaurant/Bistro offered fresh, professionally cooked food at reasonable prices. Finally, beautiful artwork and western sculptures were scattered throughout the hallways. Truly, it was a place of hope and healing. What a gift this place was.

Family and friends joined us that night. We gathered together, in a semi-circle around Karen's bed. A friend prayed. While everyone was there, a medical team came in to examine Karen's eyes, as melanoma often lurks in that area of the body.

As I watched Karen go through the exam, I felt agitated and protective. There she was – my wife, in a hospital bed, recovering from brain surgery – having her eyes examined for the possible presence of melanoma behind them. These specialists treated her with utmost respect, but I still found myself thinking, "Why are you touching her? Be gentle with her, please." I could barely control myself.

It would be the first of many, many exams trying to anticipate melanoma's movement and schemes in Karen's body, so she and the physicians could counter-attack. Thankfully, Karen's eyes were clear. No sign of melanoma there.

Eventually, everyone but me went home. Out came the hide-a-bed, surprisingly comfortable. Karen and I talked for a few minutes, then we both fell asleep and, except for the periodic, mandatory vitals checks by the nurse, and blood draws by phlebotomists, the only distractions in the room through the night were the IV pump, BP monitor, and dim night light.

The next morning, Drs. Jensen and Samlowski appeared during their morning rounds. I soon learned what "rounds" meant. In a teaching hospital, the attending physicians go from room to room, checking in on patients and dialoguing with their students (interns, residents and fellows) along the way. After the physician has given the student-MDs an overview in the hospital hallway, they enter the patient's room and, if possible, interact with the patient or caregiver. This morning, Karen was quite alert, and she actively engaged anyone who came through the door. It was part of her inquisitive nature. I was immensely proud of her.

I began to learn the "inside baseball" story of the medical world. Who was who? When and how to ask questions? How to advocate for Karen, and get a proactive, cooperative response, while not acting as a jerk? How to anticipate what came next? Drs. Jensen and Samlowski seemed to appreciate this approach, too. They always invited questions. "I see you have your list of questions, Sterling. Go ahead."

Dr. Jensen was pleased with Karen's neurological response and overall appearance, this just a few days after the surgery. Dr. Samlowski repeated his ideal timeline: appointment with him, radiation, and then immune-therapy (not traditional chemotherapy) starting afterward. Clearly, this was a marathon, not a sprint.

At the Huntsman, nurse practitioners (NPs) are the primary interface between the physicians and patients. They, along with the RNs, MAs, and other support staff, make the whole process work. The next morning, a nurse practitioner came by our room, telling us Karen had made such good progress that she would be discharged that afternoon. That was fantastic news. Without a doubt, home is the preferred place to recover. The discharge process takes time, as there are papers to sign, physician's care instructions to discuss, emergency phone numbers to obtain, and printed prescriptions to carry back to Walgreens.

Equally important, there was a detailed schedule for Karen's next appointment, a lengthy consultation with Dr. Samlowski. Like a bicycle wheel, he would be the hub, the central coordination point for all Karen's care. The other Huntsman staff was the spokes.

Hospital rules required that a staff person move Karen down to the lobby in a wheelchair. I walked beside her, arms full of all our stuff, until we got to the lobby, and then I ran to get the car.

Off we went, heading home.

Earlier, three of my children had said their good-byes and returned to college in Southern California, this after they were confident that their mother was on the mend and would soon head home to recover. They would find friends and supportive professors there, minus the constant reminder of their mom's illness.

Physician's prescriptions in hand, Karen and I went over to a Walgreens that night to get the medicines. Silly me! What was I thinking? "Karen, do you want to go for a little drive, just like old times?" By the time we got there, it was 8 p.m. In addition, a swamped pharmacy, stressed staff, long prescription turn-around time, and exhausted wife, taught me a big lesson: Don't do that again!

In the future, I enlisted neighbors to sit with her while I ran to get medications or food, especially when Karen was on the front end of recovery from a medical procedure. Eventually, I figured out how to make things work. I actually became good at it. Along the way, I learned to love my wife in a whole new way.

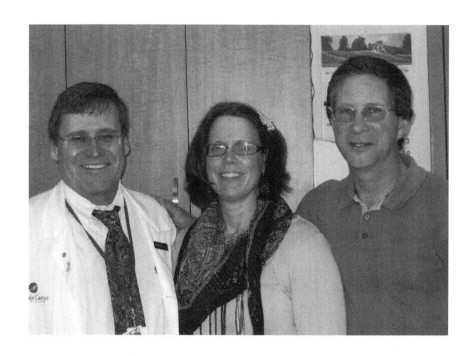

Dr. Samlowski, Karen, Sterling

~6~

Statistics in the Rear-View Mirror

Confident that Karen was making solid progress, I arranged for my mother-in-law to fly up to Salt Lake for a week so I could continue my work, a job where I traveled out-of-town once a month on contract for the FAA.

"Life is what happens when you are busy making other plans," said a well-known contemporary musician/philosopher. Among other "happenings", a church friend and I had a trip to India planned since early summer, the two of us scouting out ways our local Utah church could support Indian pastors. It was my chance to return to India after twenty-four years.

After Karen's discharge from the Huntsman, I went back and forth in my mind for several weeks about whether I should go on this trip or not. At the time, such internal debate seemed reasonable to me. In hindsight, it was crazy, idealistic thinking.

Life happened; reality set in. Karen had just gone through brain surgery, and radiation was on the horizon. She had melanoma cells in two major parts of her body and I was considering flying half way around the world for a non-essential missions trip? What was I thinking?

As the seriousness of her illness caught up with me, I pulled the plug on the trip with little regret. For the next twelve months, I limited my contract business travel to five days per month, and then only if another older adult – family or friend – would be in the house with Karen.

Fortunately, post-surgery, Karen was up, eating normally, running around town with my mother-in-law, and when I returned, with me. We were grateful; she was one strong woman. Apart from the surgery scar, one had to wonder: Did she really have melanoma?

November 7, 2006 came and with it our first appointment at the Huntsman Cancer Hospital. We walked the Huntsman's long outpatient hall to Clinic 2D, whose staff specialized in several types of cancers, including melanoma. A medical assistant took Karen's vitals and led us into a large exam room, making the ones in most community health clinics look like closets.

The reason was soon clear. At the appointment time, in walked Julie, nurse practitioner (NP), a registered nurse (RN) but with much more training and experience. Later we would learn that NPs play a critical role in cancer hospitals such as the Huntsman, providing vital care and communication between the oncologists, patients, caregivers, pharmacies, and other staff in the building. Julie spent thirty minutes with Karen before Dr. Samlowski appeared in the exam room.

Today staff would set the frame around the picture, creating a comprehensive history of Karen Allene Swan: lifestyle and diet; family and symptom history; medical care up to this point; and a complete, thorough physical exam, far more extensive than ever before. Julie asked questions rapid fire; it never let up.

Karen, wearing one of those revealing hospital "gowns," was essentially naked. This was intentional. Julie had Karen stand up, and then she carefully, respectfully, observed every square inch of her body, looking for any telltale signs of moles or discolored skin. On Karen's skin surface, everything seemed normal.

Finally done with the data gathering and physical exam, Julie left the room to consult with Dr. Samlowski. While we were alone, Karen looked at me and said, "I have never had such a thorough physical exam in all my life, especially stark naked!"

Soon, there was a rapid knock at the door. It opened and in walked four Huntsman staff: Dr. Samlowski, Julie, an RN, and a Licensed Clinic Social Worker (LCSW). Four staff for one patient! Impressive. This became the norm; cancer is a fierce foe, and to beat it back requires many resources, minds, and skills. At the Huntsman Hospital, this resource commitment was typical. They threw everything they could into the battle, made possible in part by the ongoing generosity of Jon Huntsman, Sr., who gave the HCH tens of millions of dollars of his own money to provide a holistic-care experience for patients and their families.

We knew Dr. Samlowski and Julie, but who were the others? The nurse was there to take notes and execute the oncologist's orders, while the social worker could help us navigate the cancer journey's emotional challenges, that is, if we wanted the help.

Before any serious conversation started, I pulled out a vintage cassette tape recorder and asked Dr. Samlowski if I could tape the appointment. After the group had a laugh about the retro technology, he said, "Yes", and I pressed Record. He and his staff stood, while Karen and I sat together facing them, on a small sofa ideally provided for just these sorts of situations.

Dr. Samlowski recapped what he knew so far about Karen's situation, drawn from conversations with Dr. Jensen (the neurosurgeon), the biopsy, Julie's preliminary exam, and his many years of experience fighting melanoma.

"Melanoma typically starts on the skin surface, but not always," he explained. "This is why Julie gave you a full body exam. In a small percentage of cases, it starts inside the body, where the sun never shines. This appears true for you. This type cancer also likes to metastasize, or spread, to the brain. When that happens, we call it Stage IV, the highest level.

"Your level.

"The tumor in your right temporal lobe has probably grown there for many months. Historically, survival rates for Stage IV melanoma are often less than one year. I want to emphasize that these statistics are backward looking, like looking in the rear-view mirror of a car. Amazing advances in treating melanoma are becoming available as we speak, leading to options I will discuss with you today that could extend your life for many years."

With those words, Karen started to weep. It was a hard message to hear. As I looked around the room at these four faces, I realized that it was a hard message for them to deliver as well. They were all somber. Some looked down at the ground.

"This is a very serious disease, and it could very well take your life," added Dr. Samlowski, "but you can fight it if you want."

If she wanted to fight?

I already knew the answer to that. Karen's personality wired her to meet challenges head-on; that determination was a key element in her pushing back on cancer for so long. When it came to will-to-live, the doctor was speaking to the right woman.

Karen and I asked follow-up questions, at least the ones we knew how to ask. A lengthy discussion followed. Then, it was decision time: What did she want?

Think about it at home?

Decide now?

Karen was a fighter; she was all in.

"I want to start treatment immediately."

So it would be.

Dr. Samlowski explained that Karen would get targeted, computer-controlled brain radiation as soon as possible – the second treatment component essential for stabilizing the brain – then start an intense, infusion-based drug treatment regimen after the New Year, assuming her brain had recovered enough by that time to withstand the stress. He and Julie would coordinate all of Karen's care with other oncologists and staff in the months ahead.

What about her lung tumor? That one, about the size of a golf ball near the pulmonary artery, would require a biopsy, then removal, but not right away. Everything in its time! The pressing need was to continue stabilizing the brain.

While no one wants to get cancer, the year 2006 was right on the cusp of some exciting, groundbreaking drug treatments for melanoma. In addition, the Huntsman, a national cancer center, was at the forefront of conducting clinical trials on these new drugs. In the midst of some very ominous storm clouds, we could see rays of hope.

As the medical staff left, John Conley, the social worker, remained. He gave us a human-flavored perspective on where things were at (neurological issues, his specialty), and the looming psychological battle with cancer. Over time, Dr. Conley would become one of our best friends, often joining Karen and I during appointments with oncologists, and follow-up sessions after scans when we would get results from brain MRIs. We increasingly leaned on John to give us "the rest of the story," and we would call on him often, even after normal office hours.

Our appointment was finally over. The information and implications had come at us fast and furious. I felt like we had taken a drink out of a fire hose. After a stop at the Clinic's front desk to schedule an appointment with the radiation oncologist – the physician who would walk us through the radiation treatment process later in the month – we took an elevator down to parking and headed home, home to a new normal.

Clearly, not only was my India trip impossible, I had a new job, full-time advocate and caregiver for my wife as she dealt with the scourge of Stage IV melanoma cancer.

~7~

First Radiation

Anyone who has gone to a dentist has likely received radiation, x-rays to spot teeth cavities and other issues. It is low dose and rather harmless, so much so that dental assistants typically handle the scan procedure. Radiation designed to treat cancer is in another league. In early November 2006, we would soon understand why radiating tumor cells is a medical specialization all by itself.

Cancer radiation, especially of the brain, has come a long way since the days where the only option was to bathe the tumor area with multiple doses of low-level radiation. Unfortunately, radiation does not discriminate between "good" and "bad" cells; the less precise the radiation beam, the greater potential damage to healthy tissue – brain, lung, abdomen, etc. While cancer cells are killed, side effects can complicate or impair a patient's complex biological system in other areas, such as memory, breathing, or bladder control just to name a few.

In recent years, advanced computer technology and scan options have merged, providing oncologists with a powerful new tool: stereotactic radiosurgery, or SRS for short. Dr. Shrieve, another experienced HCH physician (and the ever-present resident or fellow, plus nurse), met with Karen and I in early November for an hour-long consultation. During this overview appointment, Dr. Shrieve explained in detail both whole brain and SRS radiation options, how these two treatment strategies might apply in Karen's situation, and finally, his recommendation. Once again, on a medical/technical level, it was fascinating stuff. On a personal level, I so wished it was not Karen's brain that was the center of attention.

Here were the essential details: up to 70% of a tumor comes out at surgery, around 20% is killed via radiation, and ideally, the remaining 10% is either killed or controlled by drug treatments. This last part, the 10%, is particularly difficult with brain cancers because of what medicine calls the blood/brain barrier, where the brain's biology normally "walls off" many drugs from getting to the disease.

Like most things in life, there are trade-offs between whole brain and SRS radiations. Dr. Shrieve favored SRS in Karen's case because the brain target area was largely defined; raising the likelihood of killing more cancer cells without damaging good ones.

How does a patient prepare for SRS? What are the common and potential side effects? Once we had that information on the table, Karen decided on the spot: I want SRS. She had a good mind, outgoing personality, and a love for life, qualities she did not want to risk losing in the effort to kill off melanoma tumor cells. Her desire was to live life as much as possible, not just exist.

The decision made, we had one final hurdle, verifying Blue Cross would pay for the stereotactic radiosurgery, which costs tens of thousands of dollars "retail," compared to just a few thousand dollars for a full treatment of whole brain radiation. How to get this approved? My insurance expected a written justification of medical necessity from Dr. Shrieve. Rumor was that they rarely declined SRS procedures recommended by the Huntsman, but they still wanted to see the detailed explanation. Approval in hand, we could proceed.

*****

SRS is an advanced, computer-controlled radiation machine that oncologists use to radiate a tumor area – ideally a perimeter area around the tumor – to kill off tumor cells. Sometimes SRS follows a surgery, or in lieu of it. SRS is part radiation, part physics, part hope, in that the tangerine-size target, called a tumor cavity, is inside Karen's brain. It is like trying to hit a seed inside an orange, while at the same time, impacting as little of the surrounding "tissue" as possible.

How is this possible? A combination of astounding technology, brilliant medical minds, and steel-like courage on the patient's part come together to attempt a good outcome. A few years ago, this technology did not exist. Now, it could potentially extend Karen's life for many years. At the center of all this was a human being whose courage seemed boundless. She and I agreed that the many prayers offered up for her during the long cancer journey reinforced this innate strength. She sensed it.

Here is how the drama would play out. First, an MRI brain scan defines the tumor target. Next, physicians use those tumor coordinates to program the radiation machine's computer. Preparations complete, Karen is brought in, laid on a full-length table, face up, with her body, particularly head, carefully restrained. Finally, radiation technicians run the computer program, which guides a large radiation generation "head", mounted on an articulating arm, to rotating around her brain, zeroing in on the target.

To solve the challenge of reaching the tumor tissue without damaging too many good cells, the SRS software directed the radiation generator to create thousands of small slices that, collectively, would follow along the tumor's parameter, slicing around Karen's brain. Like a paper hand fan, wide at one end, narrowing at the other, these slices, in total, added up to a full radiation treatment. Unlike whole brain radiation, SRS was just a one-time treatment event, targeting only the offending tissue. In theory at least, the technology spared life-governing tissue while killing off the malignant tissue.

One obvious problem: How would Karen's head get bolted to the table, since absolute precision was essential, and any movement, even by fractions of millimeters, would subject her brain to unnecessary radiation or miss the target area? The solution to this restraint requirement was to bolt a halo, made of lightweight metal, to her skull, and then attach that halo to the table.

Bolt?

Yes. Dr. Shrieve himself would attach the halo the morning of the procedure, placed on Karen's head like a ¼" thick headband just above her eyebrows, encircling her head. Four points on Karen's scalp, equidistant from each other, would be numbed, and then the halo attached using four pointed screws that bore into her skin, ultimately resting on her skull.

It is a gruesome picture; there is no way of minimizing the difficulty of some of these treatment choices. This part of the procedure preparation was not only difficult for the patient; it is also tough on the staff. That is why the radiation oncologist himself did the halo placement.

*****

November 22, 2006 – SRS procedure day

As this was Karen's first SRS treatment, everything – a targeting MRI the day before, wearing the restraining halo, worrying about side effects of body and personality impairment – was new. It is not unusual for patients to take Valium starting the day before the SRS procedure. Karen was calm enough this time around not to need a relaxant. Me? I forced all my emotions down, way down. Eventually, that holding tank overflowed years later.

We checked into the Huntsman outpatient radiation clinic the morning of the SRS procedure. Nurse practitioners, registered nurses, and medical assistants were ready for Karen, not just with a precise medical protocol, but many creature comforts, including snacks, juice, water, warm blankets, and many, many words of encouragement. The Huntsman works hard at selecting staff that are not only technically competent, but decent human beings, emotionally intelligent. It showed; kindness contributes to health and healing. Staff asked if Karen wanted music playing in her headphones during the procedure. She chose classical.

The halo placement was next. This was the only time in seven years of Karen's care that staff "invited" me not to be in the room when Karen underwent preparation for a procedure. I judged it wisdom from experience. So I waited down the hall, as Dr. Shrieve and his colleagues did their necessary work.

Once the halo was attached to Karen's skull, I had one final chance to see her. Staff led me into the prep room…and there she was, somber, hurting, resigned, yet determined. "That Look" nearly killed me. After a quick kiss, staff wheeled her to the radiation room.

"Allow about an hour," they said. I headed up to the 6th floor's Pointe restaurant for some breakfast. It was a helpful refuge from all the serious treatment going on several floors below me.

As promised, the procedure only took an hour. Karen's nurse walked directly towards me as I sat in the waiting area, providing a concise update.

"The procedure went well," she said. "Karen is in an exam room. The halo is off. You can join her. After one of my MA colleagues helps her gets dressed, I will come back in to explain what happens from this point on."

What happens when a confined space is heated up, such as water in a teakettle? Pressure builds. Since Karen's brain had just been "heated up" by the radiation, a discharge nurse told us to expect a number of common side effects, like headaches, dizziness, and complications to overall body and personality functions associated with that particular brain lobe.

Steroids are the go-to drugs to reduce this swelling, which is the prescription we were given; strong dose up front to calm her brain, that vital organ, with a decreasing taper regimen for the weeks ahead. What about complications? I was given a 24-hour Huntsman number to call. As for a follow-up MRI, and appointment with Dr. Jensen, both were scheduled in a month, the middle of December. Merry Christmas!

While Karen looked better minus that halo, she was exhausted, so staff wheeled her out into the HCH lobby while I went to get the car. Our drive home was one of those surreal moments. Karen just had her brain radiated, yet apart from two visible, bruised areas on her forehead, an outsider would never have known. The world kept spinning, just as it always did, and we kept heading down a roaring river in our little Swan boat.

For Karen, steroids were a blessing and a curse. While they probably helped reduce the swelling in her brain, they also caused immediate side effects, most noticeably extreme agitation, which led to sleeplessness, which meant frequent verbal battles between us, to the point where life at home sometimes became very difficult. I felt I was walking on eggshells; Neil, almost fourteen, tried to play things "calm and cool" as much as he possibly could.

In addition, tinkering with the brain causes all sorts of unintended consequences, such as amplifying personality strengths and weaknesses, drifting away from some old friends, hobbies, and attitudes, while acquiring new ones. Most personal for me, Karen's brain radiation changed the dynamic of our marriage relationship.

What caused these changes? Was it the removal of the right temporal lobe? Radiation? Brain trauma? I suspect my children saw it. I definitely did, as I was with Karen almost all the time. Did Karen perceive the changes she was experiencing? I am not sure, and I did not ask. What was the point? Fortunately, only Neil was living at home full-time, and thankfully, he was in a very supportive school during weekdays. Fact was, there was nothing we, or medicine, could do about it. The brain remains a mysterious organ.

※※※※※

Come December, a blizzard of bills from various medical providers started filling my mailbox, pages and pages of them. In all the years of raising children, with their occasional medical issues, I had never seen such bill volume and complexity.

I quickly become an expert in billing codes, my written insurance contract, "medical necessity" determinations, provider and insurance customer service, and steps to correct errors. As my sister, Colleen, noted some years later, my personality seemed well-suited for this aspect of Karen's medical journey, as I considered staying on top of all the bills a personal challenge. Turning my back on this "job" for even a week would have swamped me. I handled all the bills, not Karen. I did not even discuss them with her, as she had the greater challenge, staying focused on the cancer fight and living life.

Providentially, I had a high-quality PPO health care plan that allowed Karen to get outstanding treatment at the Huntsman, with only expensive procedures like SRS requiring prior approval. In addition, I had a retirement income from my career with the FAA, and occasional generous gifts from people that allowed me to pay off most of the University of Utah Health Care bills every month. Handling the myriad of medical bill issues was one of the ways I learned to serve my wife.

By the time Thanksgiving rolled around, we had tapered Karen's steroid dose enough that the personality disruptions were few and far between, which meant a meaningful, low-key holiday. A few weeks later, my three oldest children returned from college. The Christmas season was spooling up, Karen was recovering nicely from her radiation, and we started hitting our stride again as a family, albeit with new expectations. It was an interlude between storms, a break we all needed.

~8~

Woman in the Bed

Over the years, I kidded Karen about her amazing stamina, including suggesting that she probably rowed across the Atlantic ocean from The Old Country, in a single person canoe, with an oar in one hand and a cup of coffee in the other.

My absurd humor aside, her physical and emotional strength would prove essential as we entered 2007. After looking at December's MRI, Dr. Jensen concluded that Karen's brain was stable enough to continue with more general melanoma treatment. With that green light, we met with Dr. Samlowski in early January, where he spelled out what was next in the treatment regimen: biotherapy, using three drugs that would possibly work in her brain, and more likely, throughout the rest of her body.

The source of Karen's melanoma, right lung or someplace else, no longer mattered; it had metastasized to her brain, requiring a full counter-attack. Dr. Samlowski's recommended three-drug melanoma "cocktail" (Interferon, Interleukin – IL2, Temodar) was designed to stimulate Karen's immune system and thereby provoke her body to attack the melanoma cells more aggressively. Old-school chemotherapy would not only kill "bad" cancer cells but many "good" cells as well, causing serious, life-threatening complications. This new bio-chemo therapy took a different approach by enlisting one's own immune system to fight the disease.

As with anything in life, there is no free lunch; everything has a cost, obvious or hidden. Stimulating Karen's immune system would stress her whole body, especially weakest areas, so Dr. Samlowski arranged for an evaluation of her overall cardiovascular condition before one milliliter of medicine dripped into her veins. To assess this, Huntsman staff put her on a treadmill and carefully measured her lung capacity, heart rate, and a host of other factors, including a battery of blood labs. Could she handle the side effects these drugs will likely produce in her body? Is she truly physically strong enough? There was no point subjecting Karen to harsh chemicals if the results were rapid impairment, trauma, or death.

Karen easily passed the physical assessment. Maybe it was the coffee?

Because of toxicity, cancer-fighting medicines are often administered via IV. So it would be with Karen. Typically, patients receive chemo (short for chemical) therapy treatment in an outpatient setting, i.e., in a clinic.

Not with this cocktail. Because of well-known side effects, Karen would receive these drugs in-patient, over a period of 96 straight hours, under the watchful eye of Dr. Samlowski and a staff of nurses and support staff. Some staff said that the first 24 hours of continuous infusion with these powerful drugs was like getting hit by a freight train. The body was pummeled.

I thought this brutal-sounding imagery seemed a bit overplayed, perhaps even scaring off some patients. Not with Karen. She did not hesitate; she was all in. It was her mindset throughout the 7½-year journey fighting cancer. Her decision made, staff started the ball rolling behind the scenes so that Karen could get the infusion therapy towards the end of January.

*****

The "new normal" of the Swan world seemed like a dream. To look at Karen, one would never know she had cancer. She had a beautiful, full head of hair; we regularly walked the neighborhood and hiked in the local mountains; she drove our car by herself; she ate normally; and maintained her hobbies, including skiing, snowshoeing, bicycle riding, cooking, and sewing. We regularly attended a local church, and she had many friends. Yet, subconsciously, I think all six of us knew that Karen's health, and life, were fleeting. This melanoma cancer was a tenacious foe, and the harshness of the treatments merely served to underscore the seriousness of the battle.

Though each of my children responded to their mother's illness in a unique way, just by the nature of things, we were all in this together. At the same time, Karen's cancer diagnosis had spiked genuine concern from extended family and friends, but as the months clicked by, people went on with their lives.

Looking back, I now understand that humans – spouse, children, extended family, friends, and Huntsman staff – can only do so much. There were other forces at work, spiritual ones that sustained us behind the scenes.

Then, I was largely clueless.

Now, I get it.

*****

On a Monday in late January, Treatment Day 1 had arrived. Karen and I took an elevator up to the Huntsman's fifth floor, one of two in-patient levels, and there met intake staff that ushered Karen and me to her private room, exactly like the one she had been in last October. Bernadette Bitters, a nurse practitioner, popped into our room and talked us through the upcoming treatment marathon. Procedures were explained; paperwork signed.

"Karen, do you have an Advanced Medical Directive," she asked? A what? Karen did not, so Bernadette gave us a Utah state-sanctioned copy, encouraged a candid discussion about the form's options, and strongly recommended its completion, including a non-family witness signature, before treatment began later on that afternoon.

Really?

Before?

In addition, she explained that cancer-treatment-certified nurses would oversee Karen's care 24/7, with about a 5/1 patient to staff ratio. Karen would soon change into comfortable hospital clothing, she could order dinner from an extensive menu, there was a DVD library where we could borrow films to watch within the room, and for those that appreciated the outdoors, there was a large courtyard behind the hospital that looked east, into the mountains. It was a good news/bad news briefing. This was all brand new stuff.

"Dr. Samlowski will come to your room later on this afternoon to check in on you and answer any last-minute questions," said Bernadette. "Until then, relax. Once the infusion starts, Karen's body will determine how things play out."

Dr. Samlowski did drop by, with his professional, yet disarming personality that Karen and I had grown to value the last three months. After some light-hearted talk, he reiterated that while Karen's body might react to the powerful medicines, she should push through it if at all possible. The FDA only allowed 96 hours of elapsed time from the moment the infusion started, no matter whether the meds were dripping into her or not.

"What questions do you have, Sterling?" said the doctor. He was getting used to me. I had a few, which he addressed, and then he was gone.

A few minutes later, several nurses appeared, pushing a cart with several small plastic bags of fluid that I surmised were the meds. They checked and double checked the physician's orders, Karen's name on the bags, the volume in the bags, and then went about setting the infusion pumps to properly drip two of Karen's meds.

Their checks complete, I asked to see what they were doing. "Educate me, please." They did. I wanted to own Karen's care; information was power.

Finally, it was time. A nurse double-checked an in-line electronic monitor responsible for regulating drug volume, grasped a valve, and moved a small roller blocking the line, which then released Interleukin and Interferon into Karen's body. Temodar, the third drug in this cocktail, was given orally.

With that, the nurses left.

The sun sets early in January; night came quickly and all was well, or so it seemed. Neither of us was interest in watching TV. I read. Karen rested in her hospital bed, back raised so she could look around. We talked, about the day's events, the cancer journey so far, our children, and what might take place over the next few hours. But with all the intense activity earlier in the day, we both mainly chilled out.

Occasionally, a nurse, MA or phlebotomist popped in, checking vitals, drip lines, or drawing blood for lab tests. Confident that things were finally on autopilot, with no sound of an approaching freight train, I headed up to the sixth floor to grab some dinner at the Huntsman's Bistro, open late to serve family and friends.

The full-length couch in Karen's room converted into a hide-a-bed, so when I returned from dinner, I unfolded the bed and made it with the clean sheets, blanket, and pillow provided by the staff. By then, Karen was fading quickly, so I sat next to her, holding her hand while singing a few lines from one of her favorite hymns.

My wife was finally asleep, and as my head hit the pillow, I was out within seconds.

Then...Crash!

It was 11 p.m.

The freight train had just plowed into Karen.

I awoke with a start, to lights on, two nurses in the room, and Karen hunched over in her bed, gasping for breath. One of the nurses sat on the hospital bed right behind Karen, holding her close, rubbing her back, encouraging her to breathe slowly, deliberately. Although she had asthma, I had never seen Karen gasping so hard for air as I did at that moment. The other nurse was closely monitoring vitals and paging the Resident–On-Call. I stood silently in a dark corner, shocked and distressed at the drama playing out before my eyes. I wanted so much to protect Karen, but there was nothing I could do. Nothing. It was one of the worst feelings I have ever had.

A doctor soon appeared. She was not a melanoma oncologist, rather, a resident, with 2-4 years of experience beyond medical school, still in training, working the overnight shift in this complex cancer hospital. When patients experience trauma, residents are often on the front lines. The more experienced, attending staff oncologists are just a phone call away, but on this particular night, apparently this resident was so concerned that Karen would lose consciousness that she decided to suspend infusion of Interleukin, the harshest of the three meds. It was a real-time decision, based on Karen's clear distress, and I respected the call.

To my great relief, Karen's breathing started returning to normal after about fifteen minutes. Someone dimmed the lights, a nurse remained at her bedside, and as I sat in a chair next to her, holding her hand, she fell asleep. The train had crashed into her; now she needed to recover.

Slumped in the chair, I also fell back asleep.

With sunrise came the thought: Was that a nightmare? Did Karen really go through that horrific trauma last night?

It was no dream.

Karen, awake, exhausted but hungry, ordered a vegetable omelet off the menu. She gobbled it down as soon as it was delivered. In between bites, we talked. She remembered very little of the previous night's breathing trauma; it was all a blur to her. A report of the complications had reached Dr. Samlowski, who was in Karen's room, at her bedside again, first thing.

He had already talked with the resident and floor nurses about Karen's reaction to the Interleukin (IL2); now, he wanted Karen's and my perspectives on the incident, and how she was feeling eight hours later. "This was an expected reaction to the IL2," he said. "Many patients experience it to one degree or another. "

Although genuinely concerned for Karen's wellbeing, rather than suspending the IL2 treatment, I sensed that Dr. Samlowski much preferred that the resident had used other options to deal with Karen's breathing difficulties, strategies that might have been able to mitigate the drug's side effects. Eight hours of treatment had been lost so far, and he strongly recommended that Karen restart the infusion as soon as possible, guaranteeing that he would personally respond if Karen experienced other complications. Finally, he also ordered asthma medication doses for Karen, delivered throughout the day by a staff person who specialized in that sort of in-patient treatment.

With light streaming in the window, a reasonable rest, good food in her stomach, and clarity about what she was up against, Karen, the courageous woman, readily agreed to the restart. Within minutes, a nurse had opened the valve on the drip line containing that powerful drug. I asked Dr. Samlowski if these "lost hours" could somehow be made up.

"No," he said. "Federal Drug Administration (FDA) rules prohibited it."

So it goes.

Karen was sobered by the previous night's trauma, yet hardly downcast. Determined to stare down this cancer enemy, she was willing to push through the nearly 80 hours ahead. To change the dance a bit, she got out of bed and, with an MA's help, dragged the two poles over to the room couch so we could sit together, hold hands, talk, and yes, even laugh.

*****

There was a knock at the door.

In walked a group of staff oncologists, residents, and fellows doing rounds. The senior oncologist had briefed his student-colleagues about Karen's status in the hallway before entering the room, and now they wanted to get our take on how her treatment was going. Karen talked a bit, but as would become common in the months and years ahead, she deferred to me to answer most of their questions and describe what had happened the night before. I jumped in with a detailed explanation, seasoning my facts with some patient advocacy.

Because time was at a premium with this on-the-job training class, there was no small talk; as quickly as they had arrived, they were gone, to the next patient, who was likely undergoing treatment for a different type of cancer. After their departure, Karen and I continued our random, low-key conversations, even as a steady stream of nurses, MA's, and phlebotomists came into the room doing their jobs, part of a complex web of medical staff committed to Karen's wellbeing.

A new person appeared in our room, a staff nutritionist. It was her job to monitor Karen's nutritional needs while she was inpatient, making sure that Karen was getting a balanced diet, even when she was not all that hungry. How would that work? If Karen got to the point where she was not interested in eating food by mouth, this nutritionist would create a liquid diet, hang it on one of the poles, and drip the nutrient into one of Karen's vein. It was a high-tech smoothie. Regular blood draws and urine samples would tell the nutritional tale; behind the scenes, this woman was carefully monitoring Karen's overall health.

Bernadette, NP, popped in again, and by that time, Karen was ready to get back into her hospital bed, so the three of us worked together to make that happen. Once settled, Bernadette asked Karen to explain what she remembered from last night. She also asked me. Then she added some experience-based perspective on what Karen could expect in the hours ahead: perhaps one or two more impact "punches" from IL2, followed by increased drowsiness, also a "normal" IL2 side effect.

One of my constant companions was an 8 ½ x 11-inch notebook. Anytime Karen or I spoke with a Huntsman staff person, physician all the way down the line to MA and nutritionist, I wrote down their names, contact information, and any medical details they gave on Karen's condition, treatment to date, drugs used, and responses to questions Karen and I would ask. It became part of the historical record of Karen's care, and I often referred to it when medical staff was in the room. Capturing information not only helped Karen and I stay on top of things, it helped the staff with the myriad of details involved in her care, details that were not always spelled out in the charts or digital notes.

In the early afternoon, Karen had another bout of breathing difficulty. When I saw it coming on, I flagged the nurse sitting at a workstation just outside our door. Instantly she was in the room along with an MA, and soon, Dr. Samlowski and an asthma specialist appeared. Within minutes, Karen received a steroid via nebulizer and the breathing challenge passed.

As Bernadette had forecast, gradually Karen became more and more sleepy, even though it was just mid-afternoon. Friends and family would pop in to visit, which was a wonderful gift to Karen and I, as these folks would sit with Karen, talk for a few minutes, or if she was sleeping, quietly read. We never turned on the TV, since it was not calming.

When a friend or family member dropped in, if at all possible, I headed up to the 6th floor to get some coffee or a meal. I used to eat the part of Karen's meals that she could not finish, only to discover that sharing food was throwing off the nutritionist's calculations of her needs! How? The nutritionist was monitoring all the things that Karen ordered off the menu. If Karen ordered something, sharing part with me, the nutritionist recorded that Karen ate that entire item. Once we figured that out, I reluctantly stopped eating Karen's leftover food. I could either order my own meal off the same menu or run upstairs for a mental health break.

As the sun set Tuesday night, Karen was relaxed, and except for the times when she got poked by the phlebotomist for a blood draw, in a sleepy/dreamy state. I made phone calls, read, dozed, went to the floor's library to use the computer, and found other ways to kill time before pulling out the bed and sleeping myself.

Dr. Samlowski checked in one more time. After the night staff took over, the floor calmed down. Apart from infusion pump and monitor sounds, things were mostly quiet. While we were woken up several times during the early morning hours for blood draws, thankfully the freight train was gone. Karen had pushed past that.

Like clockwork, our hospital floor came to life the next morning. Before day staff showed up, I was able to grab a shower in an area provided for family members entirely apart from the patient's bathroom. When I returned, physician rounds had started.

Night shift nurses handed off to the day shift; the floor was getting busy. There were more lab tests and a quick visit by Dr. Samlowski. Strange, but Karen and I were settling into a routine. As predicted, Karen's appetite was dropping off; she was ordering less from the menu, so the nutrition bag got larger by the day.

Several of Karen's friends from our church dropped by that morning, which gave me the chance to run upstairs to my refuge, The Pointe Restaurant. Breakfast, always my favorite meal, meant pancakes and coffee, enjoyed slowly while I watched the Salt Lake Valley come alive and weather move through.

*****

Absent hospital staff, it was often just Karen and I, alone, in her hospital room. Although she was increasingly in a drug-induced slumber even during the day, I did not mind. Dragging one of the room's comfortable recliner chairs over next to her bed, I would camp out there for hours, reading, working on curriculum for my FAA course, writing down questions for Drs. Samlowski and Jensen, or wander out into the hall to make phone calls to my insurance company, children or friends.

More often than not, though, I would just lay my hand on Karen's body as she dozed. Sometimes I gazed at the bags of medications hanging from those poles, each drip representing Karen's desire to fight the cancer foe and live a full life. Other times, I stared at her face, her eyes closed, as she slowly breathed. She was doing something noble and courageous. Would I have done the same? If so, why?

During those private times in that cancer hospital room, sitting next to her was the most important choice I could imagine making. Staff told me that men sometimes ran away when their wives received a cancer diagnosis, filing for divorce, or withdrawing into a realm of denial. That was not true with me; something was happening in my soul, drawing me closer to my wife than ever before.

My mind would often drift, to thinking about us: how we met way back in 1979; the first two decades of our life together; our children; our experiences and adventures; and the many ways in which I let her down.

Yes, I had let her down, and God, too. For a variety of reasons, and over too many years, I had been angry with God, or probably worse yet, content with playing a religious game. Because God is invisible, Karen became an easy target. I withheld love from her and got distracted by work and other people for months at a time. Worst of all, I often just did not like her. Life and marriage had gotten quite routine and boring.

No more.

Something was about to happen.

During one of these times of reflection, after over 25 years of turbulent marriage, including frequent verbal fights and cold wars, mainly provoked by my unhappiness with life, I had an epiphany. I looked at my wife, lying in that hospital bed, every second bravely accepting strong chemicals into her body…and I saw her in a new light.

She so wanted to live, to love and be loved, to enjoy her husband, children, and even become a grandmother someday…and suddenly, dramatically, I saw myself for who I really was.

I said to myself, "She wanted love, and I had treated her poorly way too often. I judged her, withdrew love and affection, failed to apologize, and failed to lead."

I wanted to run from these thoughts, but where would I go? Facts are stubborn things. It was just Karen, in a drug-inducted slumber, me, and a spiritual spotlight shining directly into my soul.

Like fog clearing after the sun warms the air, my view of Karen, God, and myself, went through a dramatic, tectonic shift that morning in the hospital room. That woman in the bed chose to become my wife long ago, and I would be damned if I didn't serve her, care for her, love her, with all my heart. If I failed at this, I deserved to go to Hell. She was far more loyal to me than I had been to her, since my pride and laziness had kept me from making the changes necessary in my mind and heart.

No longer.

Now, with her lying in that bed day after day, it was time for me to step up and be a man, be a husband, and love her truly, the way God loved me, even during the times I did not care. Simply put, my focus in life became to esteem Karen, to love her with everything I had to give.

Little did I know that this epiphany, this profound insight gained in a hospital, not a church (and one I never shared with

Karen because I was too embarrassed to discuss it), was the first chapter of a life-shaping journey that would completely demolish and renovate my life. The changes started on that day helped me cope as Karen and I plunged down the turbulent cancer-journey river together, leading to the day of her death, and beyond. The woman in the bed was quietly teaching me what life was all about.

*****

In this midst of these deeply personal hours and days with Karen, Dr. Samlowski, the nurse practitioners, nurses, and other staff, would drift in and out of the room throughout the day, doing their jobs. There was really nothing for us to do but let the drugs do their thing and time pass, one second at a time.

Occasionally, John Conley, our social worker friend, would drop in to talk with me, and Karen, if she were able. He added a perspective that proved immensely valuable, about the personality changes we could expect from the brain surgery, radiation, and amplification of Karen's immune system. He also kept an eye on me, the caregiver, the rather invisible part of the cancer care equation.

This is not a pity-party comment, just the reality that caregivers have a unique role to play when a loved one is dealing with a long-term, chronic disease. Specifically, my personal needs we not well understood by many people, myself included. John seemed to understand me, and his services were free. What was not to like about that?

Friday morning finally arrived: Checkout Day. Karen had successfully completed her treatment, about 88 hours of infusion, not including time lost that first horrific night the train plowed into her.

It was time to go home, to heal, and to live. Karen had a zest for life that would not stop, and me, well, I had more time with her to make things right. Certainly no one could have imagined that she would have over seven roller-coaster years ahead of her, often periods of living filled with joy, hope, and spiritual insights.

Home became a great refuge, a place where children, extended family, dear friends, and even neighbors, would pop in and bring happiness to our lives. Even though I continued my one-week of travel a month, Karen was not done with infusion treatment. We learned that many melanoma patients couldn't even make it through one continuous four-day regimen; they pull the plug because the stress on the body is too great. Dr. Samlowski challenged Karen to complete as many rounds as her body and spirit could handle. Swallowing hard, she said yes, she would do another.

So when February rolled around, we were back at the Huntsman for another five-day inpatient hospital stay, this time, 96 hours of continuous infusion with no "train wreck" hindering Karen's desire to get every drop of medicine into her body. Determination aside, it did not get easier this second time around. She again experienced labored breathing within the first 12 hours, but pushed through. As time passed, she became more and more lethargic, allowing the meds to pour into her body unhindered.

I was with her 24/7, except for when children or friends would come and give me a short break. Friends were wonderful, but often they did not know how to relate to Karen's lethargy, awkwardly trying to engage her in conversation. When that did not work, they told me they felt like the visit was a waste. It most certainly was not. I learned to give instructions to visitors: sit quietly, read, pray, sing, and/or touch her. Even a few minutes with Karen is a gift to her, to me, and the entire family.

One night, after dusk, when the main staff had left and our in-patient floor quieted down, I heard an angelic sound outside our room.

A female was singing.

Well.

Very well.

The sound drifted down the in-patient corridors, overpowering the beeps of monitors, pumps, and pagers.

Her voice was powerful. Healing. Spiritual.

Intrigued, I went outside Karen's room and slowly walk towards the music's source.

It was coming from another hospital room.

When I got close to the room, I slowed way down and, while trying not to violate someone else's privacy, glanced in as I passed the open door.

What I saw was a middle-aged woman standing at the foot of a patient's bed, sheet music opened up, singing an absolutely beautiful piece of classical music.

It was one of the most amazing sights and sounds I had ever heard.

In a cancer hospital, on an in-patient floor, beauty was present. None of us – patients, caregivers, family, or staff – was alone.

*****

March came, and with it, another 96-hour in-patient infusion.

April. Ditto. Ninety-six hours.

May?

No.

"No more," Karen told Dr. Samlowski. "I cannot handle anymore."

He understood.

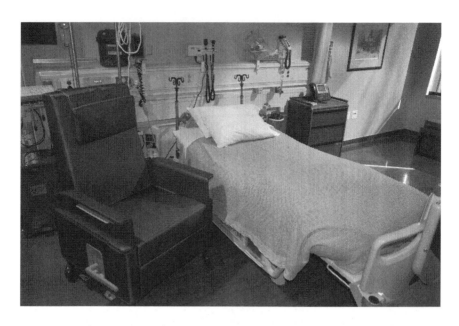

Huntsman Hospital In-patient Room

~9~

"...In Sickness and in Health..."

Our 1980 marriage vows included the traditional phrase, "in sickness and in health." Twenty-six years later, Karen was very sick. Tumors, surgery, radiation, and harsh chemicals had stressed her brain, impairing some of its normal functions. Yet, she was an extraordinarily strong woman, physically, emotionally and spiritually. She had already made incredible strides just to get to spring of 2007.

Now she was home. No more 96-hour infusion marathons. Goodbye, Interleukin.

As the staff at the Huntsman explained it, we had entered the realm of the new normal; there was no going back to our pre-October 2006 lives. Looking forward, there were many unknowns, like a turbulent river filled with whitewater, boulders and steep cliffs on both sides, challenges none of my family had ever faced before. No one takes a class, or reads a book, on what life will be like when a spouse or mother gets a life-threatening disease. All one's life prepares us for these moments, as a patient, caregiver, child, extended family member or friend. God, in his grace, also carries us, even though we often do not see it, except perhaps in hindsight.

I understand that many marriages undergo significant strain when the man is the caregiver, especially of a spouse who has a long-term, chronic disease. I certainly experienced that strain. While the "woman in the bed" epiphany had fundamentally changed my mindset and heart attitude towards Karen, the reality was that every day presented challenges that were often beyond me.

It was inevitable that my relationship with Karen started to evolve. This is actually quite normal in any marriage, but ours seemed especially so. It was just the nature of things. Looking back, I realize that Karen was doing the very best she could living life to the fullest, in the midst of having her brain – the control center of her body and personality – degraded. At the same time, I tried hard, not knowing that building mental exhaustion would put me into a funk after Karen died in 2014.

To keep our marriage from collapsing, I had to adjust. I said "sorry" more during those years than ever before, even when I did not always feel that the conflict was my fault. Peace, not "rightness," became the greater goal. I cooked more; we ate out more. I made more of an effort to support her interests and activities; my early retirement from the FAA made this possible. She had a clear shot at living life, as long as she was able.

Karen and I spent lots of time together, having fun out in nature, spending time with our children and friends, and of course, hanging out at the Huntsman, our second home. After Karen died, Neil said, "Dad, you were able to be there for mom those seven years. I think if you had put her in a care facility, she would have died within a year."

Like me, all four of my children were profoundly affected by their mom's cancer journey. Yes, their mom was physically "there," often at the house, teaching in the home school co-op, or up on the slopes, skiing, but she was absorbing one harsh treatment after another, and yes, she could die. They knew the statistics, which said most cancer patients in their mother's situation died within a year. How were they to cope?

Psychologists call this anticipatory grief. Unlike immediate grief, which occurs when a loved one dies suddenly, anticipatory grief is like the drip-drip-drip of a leaky faucet that gets worse over time.

While Neil spent his formative teen years living at home with his ill mother, my three older children were also shaped by this intense anticipation, even though college, work, AmeriCorps service, and housing away from home meant they saw her somewhat less frequently. Nonetheless, they knew she was very sick; they loved her very much. Each showed love and care based on personality and energy levels. At times, when things got too intense, they found comfort in peers and significant others, both in Utah, and distant states. I understood that.

I would like to report that extended family and friends all rallied around us and stayed engaged, but that largely did not happen. True, like most human crises, the support was initially there, but after a few months, the casserole dishes stopped coming and people went back to their own lives, leaving the Swans to a long, lonely slog. A few heroic folks did say engaged with us, year in and year out, but for most, life went on. In addition, just the word "cancer" has ominous connotations, creating generalized fears and thoughts of mortality, thoughts that can be quite troubling. Add in brain issues, and well, people get spooked.

All these reasons, and more, begin to explain why even Karen's biological family sometimes seemed baffled by the seriousness of Karen's illness, in particular, the effects the brain trauma was having on her personality, and how that influenced my marriage, shaped our children, and tested the understanding of everyone else. I believe that a woman with a cut, radiated, drugged and stressed brain that was on her feet, living life, deserved praise, honor, and patience, nothing less.

Fortunately, one of her sisters was fearless and tenacious, stepping in to serve our family in very concrete ways over the long cancer journey. Caring for a chronically ill family member, especially one living in another state, requires significant sacrifice, and reality is, each family member had to make choices on what they were going to do. Did it matter whether family or friends were Christian or not? The jury is out on that. Love shows up in many different ways.

These changing relationships were a large part of our "new normal." Words were inadequate, sentiments, rather empty, and even God's involvement in the drama, quite confusing. Actions spoke much louder than words. One day at a time, that is the best any of us could do. We would wind up repeating that bedrock spiritual truth over and over again.

*****

In this midst of all these changing family dynamics came medical complications. In late April, Karen started experiencing headaches again, above her right ear. Pain meds and steroids could not control them. An MRI scan in early May showed a significant amount of dead tissue (necrosis) in that surgery area, likely creating pressure that led to pain.

Surgery was the only answer. On May 22, 2007, Dr. Jensen opened up Karen's brain again, in the same right temporal lobe area, and removed as much of the necrosis as he could find. She spent five days at the University Hospital recovering from this brain surgery. Right after this, Karen underwent another SRS brain procedure on May 31, in the same general area, to kill off more melanoma cells that had appeared since her first SRS back in November. She had to endure the dreaded halo device and steroids after the radiation procedure was over.

Steroid side effects showed up in her almost immediately, this time with new intensity. Irritation, sleep loss, random outbursts, impulsiveness, and spikes in appetite were common. The Huntsman staff and I tinkered with the steroid dosage, hoping to find a happy medium between reducing Karen's brain swelling, and peace in the home. Achieving this difficult balance was part art, part science. These emotional and biological reactions were not Karen's "fault." Most of the time, she was only dimly aware of all that was going on.

On some days, the situation was borderline impossible, and I am confident we were given incredible amounts of strength to get us through to nightfall when I gave Karen an oral sedative, essentially knocking her out until the next morning. At times, I don't know how our relationship survived. But it did.

Once we got to summer, with warmth and opportunities for outdoor activities, Karen's brain finally started to calm down. It was a memorable couple of months together, including July, when she traveled with me to the Bay Area on one of my business trips and we played tourists in San Francisco.

At home in Sandy, Karen and I would often jump in the car and head up one of the local canyons, to hike, grab a meal at the Silver Fork Restaurant (one of our favorites), sip coffee while on Snowbird's Plaza Deck, or venture further, to one of the many National Parks in the Intermountain area. Locally, she took up bicycling with a passion, while continuing her gardening, sewing, or when she was at her best, cooking. In addition, my twin daughters spent as much time as possible with their beloved mom, including driving down to California multiple times together, primarily to hang out on the beach. It was a refuge for everyone, filled with wonderful memories.

*****

One September morning, Karen, Allene, and I were in the house, when suddenly, Karen started foaming at the mouth, her eyes rolled towards the ceiling, and she began to lose body control.

Half dragging, half carrying her into the master bedroom, I laid her on the bed, where I attempted to restrain her as she involuntarily thrashed around. While she continued to foam at the mouth and fight against me, I could hear Allene on the phone with a 911 operator, trying to explain what was going on with her mother in the midst of terrified tears.

What caused these symptoms? Like a lightening bolt on a clear summer day, this episode came out of nowhere, nearly one year into Karen's cancer journey. I was completely baffled and shocked.

Within minutes, I could hear a siren in the distance, getting closer. Next thing I knew, there were three firemen/paramedics in my bedroom, asking me details on what had happened to my wife. Their consensus: She had a seizure.

A what? Why would she have that? Why now?

By the time they had reached our home, Karen's outward physical symptoms – foaming at the mouth, eyes rolling, body flailing – had stopped. Still, she was in a psychological fog, repeating words over and over, almost completely uncooperative, and insisting that she needed to use the restroom.

I let her up to go to the bathroom, but then she locked the door and would not come out. I got a passkey and opened the door while the firemen remained in the adjoining bedroom. In the meantime, a couple of the firemen rolled a gurney into the hallway, thinking that Karen probably needed to go to the hospital.

That was not going to happen until she got dressed, something she refused to do. Fortunately, after a few more minutes, her brain settled down and she agreed to get dressed. Use the gurney? Forget it! She walked to the fire truck.

Sandy City has combination fire trucks and mini-ambulances, all in one. Once inside, a fireman asked Karen to lie down on a stretcher lashed to the floor. She would have none of it. She was going to sit up. Period. The men looked at each other and shrugged. I climbed in, snapped my seat belt, and off we went.

To where?

I told the firemen that I wanted Karen taken to the University Hospital. Could they make that happen? Yes. So there we were: three firemen, Karen, and I, traveling thirty minutes north to the

Huntsman in a Sandy City fire truck. What were they going to charge us for this "lift?" At that stage in the cancer journey, it no longer mattered to me. I had other things to worry about.

Like a homing pigeon, the fire truck pulled up to University Hospital's Emergency Vehicle Entrance. Someone opened one of the side doors and out jumped Karen, walking confidently into the admitting area. What a woman!

The ER physician agreed with the firemen that Karen probably had a seizure. Because of her recent history, she was admitted, given an MRI and steroids via IV, and a sedative for sleep. The next morning, Dr. Jensen walked into her room. He had looked at her MRI and concluded that she had experienced a simple-type seizure, something not uncommon for individuals who had suffered brain trauma.

Often seizures can be controlled, so Karen was placed on Keppra, an anti-seizure medicine. He wanted to keep her in the hospital for observation at least one more day, and if all appeared stable, released home after that.

"Dr. Jensen, when Karen had these symptoms at home yesterday morning, I had no idea what to do."

He explained: "When someone has a simple-type seizure, it typically lasts about one to two minutes. Don't restrain them. Rather, lay the person on the ground and allow them to roll without hitting anything. Or, have them sit on the ground and let the symptoms run their course. Typically, they will. In addition, calling 911 is often unnecessary, since emergency personnel cannot alleviate those symptoms.

"In Karen's case, should this happen again, call my office as soon as the symptoms have passed. If it is after hours, call the general Huntsman number and they will connect you with the Resident-On-Call.

"Finally, Karen should no longer drive a car for a while. We will decide together when she can re-start, if at all."

I brought Karen home the next day.

Once back into our home routine, an imprecise word if there ever was one, Karen asked me what had happened during the morning of her seizure. She had no memory of it other than a few fleeting elements when the symptoms were building. Most notably, she saw a red flashing light in the corner of one eye, thought it was a police car, and then everything went blank.

Among other things, I explained that three handsome firemen visited her in her bedroom, she locked herself in the bathroom for a while, and when she came out, she was dressed only in her underwear.

Initially mortified, she suddenly burst into laughter. So did I. What a trip.

Karen wanted to thank these guys for serving her, so she did what came natural, make them some food. We used to have a peach tree in our back yard that bore lots of fruit in early fall. Famous for her peach cobbler dessert, Karen decided to make these guys a huge cobbler in an aluminum foil casserole dish and bring it over to the fire station not five minutes away.

Once that cobbler masterpiece was ready, we drove to the station together, walked to the front door, and knocked. Since we had lined things up beforehand, the three firemen who had come to our home were there. Beaming, she handed them the cobbler, thanked them for coming, apologized for being a pain, and wished them well. It was a class act. Later, I wrote the city's fire chief, complimenting those three men for the way they had cared for my wife.

*****

Shortly after this seizure experience, we received a letter in the mail from University Hospital administration: Dr. Samlowski was leaving the Huntsman for an oncology position in Las Vegas.

No! Tell us it wasn't so. We were heartbroken.

We trusted and loved Dr. Samlowski. The fact that he was leaving was tough news. Now we faced the challenge of transitioning to a new oncologist. The search would take a while. In the interim, Dr. Akerley, a Huntsman lung cancer oncologist, would take over Karen's care until the Huntsman Hospital hired a new melanoma oncologist. Especially with cancer, relationships between physicians, patients, and caregivers really matter. Oh, well, so it went. We would have to trust that this change was not a random event.

Karen still had a golf-ball sized tumor in her right lung. No one had forgotten about it, but two brain surgeries, two SRS radiation treatments, and a seizure, took precedence. In the fall of 2007, her lung tumor took center stage.

A scan of her lung region showed that this tumor had not grown much. It, too, was spherical, lodged close to a key artery in her right lung. Karen and I had lengthy conversations with Dr. Akerley about whether to remove or radiate, due to the tumor's proximity to vital vessels. Did she want to risk removal if a biopsy showed that it was melanoma?

Dr. Akerley consulted with Dr. Bull, one of the Hospital's lung (thoracic) surgeons. Since the tumor was spherical, Dr. Bull believed there was good chance of a positive surgery outcome. We wondered how would they get a tissue biopsy of an object inside her lung?

Under local anesthesia, a specialist came at the tumor from Karen's back, using a small scanner to guide him as he pushed a slender needle to the tumor's edge. Once there, he carefully grabbed some of the tumor's tissue and retracted the needle.

As expected, the biopsy confirmed melanoma. With that information, Karen said, "Go for it. Get that tumor out."

All this occurred in November 2007. In addition, my contract job with the FAA was over and I said "no" to further travel. It was good timing. The world economy was about to enter the Great Recession, and Karen was in line for another surgery. I needed to be with her.

Finally, on this month, we reached a huge milestone: 13 months had passed since Karen's Stage IV cancer diagnosis. She had outlived the mortality statistics, and although we could not see around the corner, by God's grace, there was more life to live. Much more!

*****

In early December 2007, Karen and I waited in a University Hospital pre-operation surgery room; her thoracotomy (lung surgery) was scheduled in little over an hour. As in previous surgeries, we expected brief appearances by the anesthesiologist and surgeon, and then staff would wheel her to a surgery suite.

There was a knock at the door. In walked the anesthesiologist and two residents. He gave us a verbal run-down of his role in the surgery. Then, out came a small flashlight, followed by instructions for Karen tilt her head back and open her mouth wide. He performed a quick visual exam of Karen's throat & windpipe areas (larynx, trachea, etc.).

After peering into Karen's throat for a couple seconds, the physician turned off the light, rolled his small stool back a foot and, with a sly smile said, "Nice airway passages!"

We all laughed. Not only was Karen a beautiful woman, she had nice, unobstructed airways. I adopted that three-word phrase as my new, sexy way of complimenting her. No longer was it, "Wow, Karen, you look hot," or "Sweetheart, I think you are a knock-out today." Wherever we were, by ourselves or in public, I'd say with my most romantic voice, "Nice airway passages, Karen!!" It became an insider love phrase, all thanks to a physician.

*****

To get at the tumor, the surgeon had to cut out about 20% of Karen's right lung. Thankfully, that golf-ball-size tumor did not rupture; it was successfully removed, along with all residual malignant tissue he could visually see. She spent about five days in recovery, rebounding rapidly, which greatly pleased the physicians and her husband.

Following her hospital discharge, we were in for a shock. A blood test showed she had contracted a very serious staph infection, apparently while in the hospital. Oh, great. Karen survives two brain surgeries, a lung surgery, and two SRS brain radiation treatments, only to die of a bacterial infection?

Not.

University Hospital staff mobilized to help Karen fight this new foe. Because of the powerful antibiotic needed to treat a staph infection, we had to head back to the University Hospital, where they inserted a Hickman port directly into an artery next to the right side of her neck. A specialist snaked the tube connected to this port to a point close to Karen's heart, using a scanner to guide him. As he did, he noticed that she had developed a blood clot, probably a result of the recent lung surgery.

Someone was watching over Karen. Were it not for the staph infection, and the steps necessary to deal with that serious condition, this blood clot might have moved to her brain, causing serious injury or death.

Once the port was placed in Karen's upper chest, we went home, expecting a visit from a home health care nurse that afternoon. As promised, she arrived, and her job was to train me how to administer a powerful, hospital-supplied antibiotic to Karen through the port. In addition, she took daily blood samples from Karen and brought them over to the University lab so that staff could carefully monitor the bacterial level. Finally, Dr. Samlowski prescribed Coumadin, a blood thinner, to dissolve the blood clot and prevent others from forming.

It was quite a drama, with many moving pieces. After every blood draw, I received a call the next day informing me whether Karen's bacterial blood count was heading in the right direction or not. If yes, I kept the current treatment course. If not, that day's antibiotic dose was increased. The process was straightforward and deadly serious.

Two weeks after the staph bacteria first appeared, we declared victory. The germs were gone. A follow-up scan showed that the blood clot was gone, too, just in time for the 2007 Christmas holidays.

*****

Like the previous year, we kept holiday activities traditional and low-key.

Once we rolled into the New Year, Karen had a delayed Christmas present, more radiation, this time the conventional type, bathing a perimeter around the lung surgery cavity. Scans mapped the target as precisely as possible, computers were programmed, and for ten straight days she received low-dose radiation to the surgery area. Into the Huntsman radiation room she went; fifteen minutes later, we were on our way home.

Finally, her radiation treatments were over, at least for now.

~10~

Living Life to the Fullest

Karen was an optimist. She had the attitude of saying "yes" to every day, every opportunity. I was different. I tended to say "no," viewing life as more of a series of responsibilities, which trapped me into the unhealthy habit of waiting until the storms passed to engage. Of course, life never calms down. Those of us that embrace it learn to live in the midst of the challenges.

Karen was like that: Embrace! Even before the cancer diagnosis, she dove into life. After October 2006, it seemed that her brain surgeries, radiation and chemicals intensified this attitude. For example, she could not get enough of outdoor activities – skiing, snowshoeing, bicycling, hiking, gardening, get-togethers with girlfriends, especially cancer kindred spirits, church activities – more so than any time in our marriage. If I wanted to hang back, well, that was my choice, but she was all in. In addition, her senses – especially hearing, smell, and taste, sight – appeared heightened, turbocharged. What does staring death in the face do to a person? For Karen, it made her want to LIVE, to squeeze every minute out of every day; to love people and God's creation with everything she had.

Snowbird and Alta, two world-class ski areas, were up a canyon just twenty minutes from our home. Karen had taught all our children how to ski over the years, either there, or at areas up a neighboring canyon. Back in the day, getting the kids into skis and on the slopes was convenient and relatively inexpensive. Her love for skiing did not stop when she got cancer; in fact, it increased. If it was a nice day, Karen would often throw her skis in the car and head up the canyon to Alta for their "Ski Free At Three" promotion, which was two lifts, no charge, until the end of the day. In later years, Alta charged $5, then $10, for the access, but who could complain? It was a great deal.

Karen absolutely loved this. If my daughters were available, they would join her. If alone, Karen enjoyed striking up conversations with the people on her chair lift. It was an amazing opportunity for her to enjoy nature and the people who shared it with her.

For Karen, snow was good, the ocean, even better. After her lung radiation, we continued the long tradition of driving ten hours to North County San Diego, where she grew up. We stayed with her parents at their home in Vista, about ten minutes from the beach city of Oceanside and her beloved Pacific. My daughters would go with her whenever possible. So would Neil. Time permitting, they hung out in the area for weeks at a time. Snow and ocean were just what the doctor ordered for Karen's mental health.

What about the conflict between her melanoma and inevitable sun exposure at the beach or combing tide pools? Well, Karen had cancer, but cancer did not have her. She would wear full-length, high-SPF clothing, a wide brim hat, sunglasses, and layers of sunscreen. Yes, sunscreen is a hassle, but the alternative is worse. If she and my kids were going to hang out on the beach, they would always bring a large umbrella. Maybe two. Her natural photographic "eye," enhanced even more by brain complications, meant that she was constantly taking pictures, especially of sea life, water, and sunsets. Oh, the images she captured. Simply amazing!

When in Salt Lake City, the cancer journey meant acquiring new friends. It wasn't that our old friends were anti-social, just that the treatments, personality changes, marital challenges, vocabulary about the journey, etc., pushed us into a experienced-based subculture that very few people "who had not walked in our moccasins," could truly understand. Some tried; it was just very awkward.

During one of Karen's many follow-up appointments, John Conley, our Huntsman social worker, invited Karen to a support group at Salt Lake City's Cancer Wellness House (CWH), a small non-profit run for the benefit of all cancer patients, their caregivers, and children, no matter where they received treatment. John facilitated one of the patient support groups, and Karen, always game for a new experience and set of friends, started attending.

There, Karen found male and female kindred spirits who were walking a similar cancer journey path. Support groups met weekly, and Karen typically wanted to attend. Normally she drove alone, but when that wasn't possible, I brought her to the downtown Wellness Center meeting place (a remodeled house not far from the Huntsman), dropped her off, headed to Starbucks, then picked her up a couple hours later. They also had a support group for caregivers. Why I never went escapes me.

In the spring of 2008, four women – Susan, Cynthia, Tami, and Karen – hit it off. Over time, the relationships deepened. They became cancer sisters, hanging out together, not just at the weekly support group, but also at restaurant meals, coffee, outdoor activities, and occasionally, at larger dinner parties where the husbands attended. In all my years of attending church, I have never seen relationships go to such a depth, so quickly.

Apart from special events, the Cancer Sisters mostly stopped attending the Wellness House support group meetings after a couple years. Why? John Conley was no longer facilitating the group, and the Sisters had moved on in their collective cancer journeys, beyond the needs of the "newbies" that had more recently joined the group.

Cynthia and Karen grew particularly close. Although they had different types of advanced cancer and received medical care from two different cancer centers in the Valley, that did not matter. What they did have were strong Northern European personalities, similar loves (music, dance, nature, science) and to cap it off, Cynthia owned two horses, which meant the friendship was sealed.

Because of cancer-driven bone degeneration, Cynthia had lost the ability to ride her own horses, so Karen and my daughters would head out to Cynthia's home to spend the day with her and the horses. It wasn't unusual for Karen to raid our refrigerator or stop by the local supermarket, stocking up on carrots and apples for her big friends. Those were warm, wonderful times.

Not only did the Swan women become good friends with Cynthia, but Steve, Cynthia's husband, and I became fast friends, as he, too, had thrown himself fully into caring for his wife. Cynthia and Steve were one of the most generous couples I have ever met; they taught me much about how love plays out in life.

Once there were four Cancer Sisters; now there is one. Susan died first, then Karen, and seven months later, Cynthia. Tami continues her cancer battle, supported by her husband and children. It was the nature of this dreaded disease, especially at advanced stage. Every day was a gift, and friends, in a dark humor sort of way, wondered who would go first.

*****

The Cancer Wellness House staff understood that cancer patients needed social relationships with kindred spirits, and regular social/outdoor activities that would allow them to live each day to the fullest. One of their premier events was Survivors at the Summit, held at Snowbird Ski Resort's 11,000 foot Hidden Peak, the first Saturday of every August. It was a part celebration, part fundraiser, for cancer patients, families, friends, and medical staff in the area. If they had the stamina, folks could either make the hike up to Hidden Peak, or use Snowbird's renowned tram. Many chose the hike.

Transformed into a festive setting for the day, the Peak included small yellow flags with names of loved ones who were still alive or had passed, live music, short inspirational talks, and most importantly, collective joy amongst the cancer survivors and their families. While the cancer journey was brutal, none of us walked it alone.

Karen chose to hike to the top of Hidden Peak, along with my daughters and I. It was no walk in the park, but we made it, in time for the formal events, and afterward, lots and lots of hugs all around for patients, caregivers, families, and friends. What a day, on top of the world.

To cap off the day, Karen, Allene, and Amber decided to hike a short way down the mountain to catch a slow-moving chairlift for a stunning, quiet ride down to the resort's base. Feeling estranged from Karen, I took the tram down. A lot of stuff that had been piling up on my shoulders came crashing down on me that afternoon. Fortunately, my daughters were there to pick up the slack, which they did amazingly well, caring for Karen in ways I could not. Their love for their mom, on that day and many others, was clear for all to see.

After this Survivors-at-the-Summit event, Karen's interest in the Cancer Wellness House started to fade, but the friendships made there – especially her three Cancer Sisters – plus growing opportunities at the Huntsman, filled a huge need in her life, and to some degree, in mine.

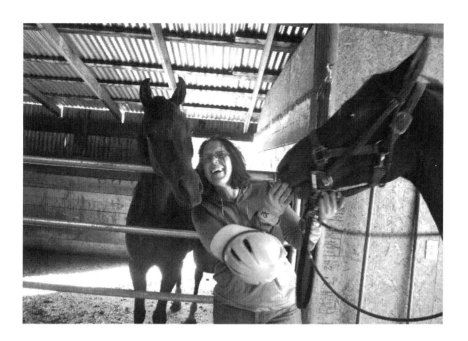

Karen at Mim's stables

~11~

HCH Wellness Center

Around the time Karen arrive at the Huntsman Cancer Hospital, management had just launched a comprehensive wellness program that had her name all over it. It dovetailed in with their philosophy of care, which went way beyond just narrowly focused medical area.

They intentionally hired competent, wonderful human beings that, together, created a supportive environment for treatment and healing. Equally important, and far beyond PR slogans, the patient as "person" was clearly valued, including the buildings themselves and an extensive wellness program that affirms the mind-body connection in life.

Along with the extensive social worker staff – I counted a dozen at one point, each specializing in a few cancers, providing services at no charge to the patients and families – the Huntsman had hired two full-time exercise specialists with master's degrees that focused on the impact of cancer on the body. These specialists ran extensive strength training programs at the Huntsman throughout the week, all no charge. In addition, there were yoga, massage, acupuncture, art, music, and other holistic-type classes that reinforced the mind-body connection in healing.

But the Wellness Center was not just about programs in a building. The two exercise specialists developed an extensive set of outdoor activities during Karen's years there. For example, it was not uncommon for a group of Huntsman cancer patients, and at least one specialist, to meet on a Saturday morning and go snowshoeing, hiking, or bicycling. Karen, and Kim, the Wellness Center's first exercise specialist, became fast friends. Because of program growth, management added Patrick, a second specialist. He became like a son, brother and mentor to Karen, someone who was known to bring Karen home from the Wellness Center activities to save me a trip. Kim and Patrick were life-giving people in Karen's life. Clearly, they loved her, and I know she loved them.

Karen enjoyed all the outdoor group activities, but to my surprise, especially took to bicycling, pursuing it from late spring through early fall. Like many Southern California kids, she had grown riding bicycles, simple Schwinn-types picked up at K-Mart. After she got cancer, I bought her a Specialized road bike that correctly fit her body's dimensions, and then she took off. Like the Alta ski experience, once the clock hit 4 p.m. (after the sun's rays were no longer a major radiation issue), Karen would often hop on her bike and ride solo for miles. She was especially fond of a 10-mile route winding around the Wilderness Area near our home.

I would often go riding with Karen, on that route and others, and with the "Wellness Center gang" during their Saturday morning summer adventures. What great memories. Had I known then what I know now, I would have participated with her in all the outdoor events, as it would have given me more time with my wife and her friends. Alas, as I also experienced with Karen's Cancer Wellness House activities, I often found myself physically and emotionally exhausted, unmotivated to join her.

Huntsman social workers explained that my experience was common in many caregivers, a nearly invisible role requiring frequently draining tasks that went on for months without let-up. For this and other reasons, I am so glad Karen threw herself into so many Wellness Center activities, as I am 100% convinced that the activities, the other patients, and the Huntsman exercise specialists, extended her life way beyond what the medical treatments alone could have done.

Finally, in many ways, Karen became the poster child for the Wellness Center. Everything they offered – art, music, exercise, massage, group activities – she tried. With gusto! Kim and Karen were even featured in a national professional journal, designed for exercise specialists like Kim and Patrick, working with the unique needs of cancer patients. It was an impressive, multi-page spread, color photos and all.

*****

Summer 2008 ended strong, with a memorable September trip to Yellowstone National Park with two of Karen's Biola college roommates and their husbands. These four long-time friends came because they loved us both and knew that cancer could soon claim her life.

The six of us spent a couple of days driving around the mountains east of my home, enjoying the fall colors, laughing a lot, playing tourist, and celebrating life. Then we drove up to Yellowstone National Park, six hours north of Salt Lake, and spent three nights in the iconic Old Faithful Inn, which is right at the doorstep of one of the world's most active volcanic areas: geysers, mud pots, billowing clouds of steam created by the boiling water, and heart-stopping beauty. It was low season in the Park, which meant that we often had the many boardwalks around the thermal areas all to ourselves. What a magical time that was, with some wonderful friends. Outdoors was a blast. Inside the 100 year-old Inn, we had plenty of time to savor meals together, talk while sipping coffee, and enjoy the live classical piano music every evening.

Whether we were in Yellowstone, or Sandy, Utah, Karen's engagement with life simply amazed me, including where she got her energy to go, go, go. For example, while I yearned for afternoon naps during our Yellowstone vacation, she wanted to go on hikes, which meant that sometimes we would part ways for hours at a time. Fortunately, while I slept, our four friends not only seem to understand this awkward dynamic, but also took steps to smooth things over.

Without these couples, and others like them, our marriage might not have survived. They became the hands and arms of God to Karen and I. There are emotional high points in my caregiver's journey with Karen during those seven years; Yellowstone in the fall of 2008 was one of them. Even now, I (mostly) smile when I think of all the memories the six of us created during those days together.

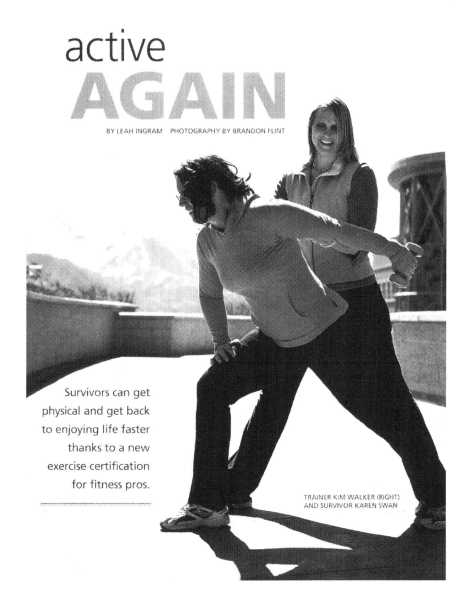

active
AGAIN

BY LEAH INGRAM   PHOTOGRAPHY BY BRANDON FLINT

Survivors can get physical and get back to enjoying life faster thanks to a new exercise certification for fitness pros.

TRAINER KIM WALKER (RIGHT) AND SURVIVOR KAREN SWAN

Huntsman Wellness Center – Karen with Kim, her trainer

~12~

It's All About Relationships

The Huntsman Cancer Hospital, thirty minutes from our Sandy house, became our second home. We made hundreds of trips to that amazing facility every year; in some years, it seemed we were there more hours in the day than anywhere else.

When Karen was first diagnosed with Stage IV melanoma, I considered getting a second opinion from an oncologist in other part of the country; in fact, the Huntsman oncologists willingly gave me the names of their colleagues at a number of large cancer centers in the West. What I concluded was that, on a medical level, the Huntsman staff favorably compared with many other facilities in the nation. Access to surgery, radiation, and medicines (even clinical trials) was largely the same, especially for Karen's type of cancer.

We knew that some of our cancer friends in other states elected to travel many hours to either a large treatment facility in their own state, or sometime to a state far away, in the hopes of finding the optimal setting that would help them beat the scourge of this dreaded disease. At one point in her journey, Karen and I did check out another cancer facility in California, thinking that maybe we would move there, and if the treatments were similar, we would be closer to family and consistently warmer weather.

We were shocked at what we found.

Like secret shoppers, we wandered around this impressive glass and steel building, checking out treatment areas, clinics, available wellness programs, patient check-in areas, restaurant/café options, and even small things like parking. Appearances aside, we felt invisible. Unnoticed. The facility was clearly understaffed, which is probably why no one ever approached us to ask if we needed help.

Even when we took the initiative to intercept a staff person to get some help, we felt that we were nothing more than a bother.

We had the answer we needed. There was no correlation between shiny new buildings and the effective delivery of holistic cancer care. The exceptional care we found at the Huntsman spoiled us; we were not going anywhere.

That "shopping" experience told us that we were in exactly the right place. The outstanding care Karen received at the Huntsman was built on relationships, on trust. Karen's medical treatments and, during the "good years," her regular follow-ups with physicians, were of course a critical piece of her survival. What could not be quantified, yet became equally critical, was that everyone at the Huntsman – from the Outpatient Support Specialist (OSS) person checking Karen in at a clinic or treatment area, to the MAs, RNs, NPs, oncologists, radiologists, clinical trial staff, Wellness Center staff, management, social workers, chaplains, even chefs at the Pointe restaurant – played a role in Karen's healing, especially her emotional wellbeing. They also played a vital role in my life as caregiver.

The staff liked us, and we, them. Karen and I made an effort to know many by name, with the unintended result that a huge "emotional bank account" was built between Mrs. & Mr. Swan, and the Huntsman staff. These "deposits" meant access when we were in crisis, support way beyond the staff's job descriptions, caring that expressed love, and candor when things got particularly difficult. This type of holistic care, of viewing the patient not primarily as a biological animal, but as a complex human being, was what the Huntsman was all about. It is why I believe we were led us to that amazing cancer facility, and why we stayed.

When Dr. Samlowski left, Drs. Akerley and Jensen became Karen's core physician team. While Dr. Akerley was not a melanoma specialist, he was caring, experienced, and straightforward, and the immediate need we had while he was Karen's primary oncologist – dealing with the tumor in her lung – was something he could address.

Over time, I learned how to speak the "oncologist" language. I would come to an appointment with a list of questions, listen carefully to the physicians (who were practicing art as well as science), and engage them. Early on, Karen and I made it clear that we were not looking for miracles. Among other things, her faith in

God produced a settled peace about mortality, which gave us the freedom to talk candidly with the physicians. They seem to deeply appreciate our outlook, as together we hashed out possible treatments, timing, and management of side effects.

Typically, when Karen came for an appointment, often the first doctor to show up in the room was a resident or fellow, alone, at least during the early years of Karen's illness. While we knew that they had to learn, the longer we were at the Huntsman, the more wearing this education process became.

Why? With each new doctor-in-training, we often had to tell much of Karen's story all over again, because there were many critical parts to her cancer treatment history. The students did not know that history, or our personalities, except for what they could read in computer-based notes or glean from their mentors. Worse, sometimes they would come in and attempt to give us bad news, say, from a recent scan.

Consequently, we learned to set boundaries. The fellows or residents could do Karen's physical exam and ask general history questions, answers I normally provided. When it came to scans or test results, or treatment options, if they made a move to reveal that information, I would stop them. Respectfully, firmly, I explained that we wanted to see the attending physician, as this information was too important to be left to someone in training.

With that, they would leave the room to summon the attending physician. Within minutes, everyone – master instructor and his students – would reappear. After a number of these uncomfortable incidents, staff put a note in Karen's bulging patient chart: Patient Requests No residents or fellows, which meant, no students coming in alone.

Even though Karen had elected to continue her melanoma care at the Huntsman after Dr. Samlowski's departure, Las Vegas was only seven hours away by car, and since the Huntsman had not yet hired a new melanoma oncologist, we maintained a long-distance relationship with this gifted physician. This meant that we had a copy of her entire Huntsman file sent down to his medical office in Vegas. Once we scheduled an appointment – often the last time slot of the day so we could have unhurried time with the doctor – Karen and I would hop in the car for a multi-day field trip.

We started this dual physician approach in the fall of 2008, and even when the Huntsman did hire a new melanoma oncologist, that physician and Dr. Samlowski knew and respected each other. Together, they provided Karen outstanding care all the way through October 2013, the last time Dr. Samlowski saw her in his office before she died.

Great challenges need collaborative effort, which meant that we kept Dr. Akerley informed of our conversations with Dr. Samlowski, and vice versa. Once the treatment options were clarified, Karen wasted no time making a decision. More often than not, if Dr. Samlowski recommended it, she would do it.

*****

As Karen visited physicians at the Huntsman and Vegas, received treatments, and even obtained prescriptions at our local Walgreens, there was another drama taking place behind the scenes. The medical insurance claims, payments, and appeals just kept on rolling in. The complicated process typically worked like this:

1) Since all of Karen's medical providers were preferred, Blue Cross looked at the billed amount (the "retail" charge), deducted a percentage based on their contract with the provider, paid the provider directly, and then sent me an Explanation of Benefits (EOB) detailing what they had decided was the total eligible amount, what they paid, and how much I owed the provider.
2) After a lag time, weeks, sometimes months, a follow-up bill from the provider would show up in my mailbox, asking for payment for the balance.
3) It was not unusual for the provider to dispute the insurance payment amount, so they would tell me they were going to rebill Blue Cross for payment reconsideration. This back-and-forth drama was like a lengthy tennis game, as both provider and insurance company had financial interests.

By now, I was used to the dozens and dozens of pages of bills and EOBs showing up monthly in my mailbox, nearly all from the University of Utah Health Care System and Blue Cross. Most of the time, Blue Cross approved all the charges for a particular date of service without pushback. Complex treatments, especially brain surgeries or professional (physician) charges for radiation treatments, were another matter. Even with prior approval, there would be billed amounts for a particular aspect of a procedure (a "line" on the claim, as the business offices called it) that would kick back to providers, typically the Huntsman, and me, the Responsible Party.

Was the right billing code used? Why was this procedure/drug/equipment necessary? There are duplicate charges for the same thing – why? This is when the billing "tennis game" got stressful for me, forcing me to redouble my efforts, start making phone calls, networking, and yes, pray.

To stay on top of things, I actively worked at understanding my insurance contract, as well as Blue Cross's medical policies underlying it, so when I called Regence, the local insurance company's Federal Employee Program (FEP) Health Benefits customer service department, I knew what I was talking about. Over time, two impressive points-of-contact, Linda and Lori, emerged within Regence's Tacoma Home Office. Whenever any complex or cumbersome issues arose claims or a prior authorization request, my first call went to one of these women.

Bills could get tangled up for the smallest reason, quickly spiraling out of control if left unaddressed. Enter Linda and Lori. Their experience and exceptional work ethic ensured that I did not fall into billing quicksand. More often than not, they had the insight to spot the problem in the claim, and then fix it while I was on the phone, or promise to call the provider's billing office directly and work it out. Amazing service! Who would have thought that my excellent insurance would be so essential when I retired from the FAA a year before Karen got sick, or that two women, in Washington state, would support Karen and I in such caring ways?

On the hospital side of the billing drama, whenever physicians ordered a procedure or treatment that required prior approval with Regence Blue Cross, Huntsman staff was all over it. Scarcely had the doctor's orders been input into the computer when they were making calls to Regence to get the thumbs-up. For anyone who has had medical treatments delayed because of roadblocks in the approval process, they will know that this team effort, from the physicians, Huntsman staff, insurance company staff, and then back to me, was exceptional and all too rare. It allowed Karen to get timely treatments and live life; and me, to avoid any more stress worrying about unpaid bills.

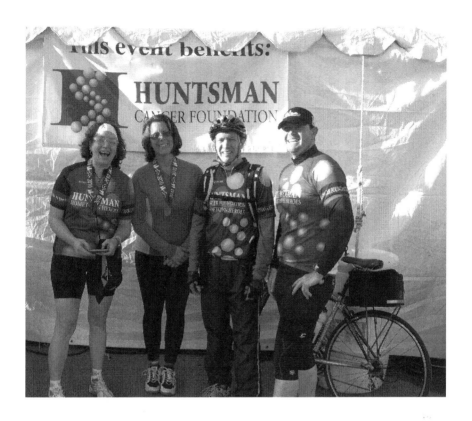

Huntsman Hometown Heroes – Finish Line – Patrick, far right

~13~

The NED-in-Brain Years

With two brain surgeries and SRS treatments to the same right frontal lobe, four rounds of in-patient immunotherapy, a lung thoracotomy followed by radiation to that area all behind her, plus enthusiastic embrace of Wellness Center programs, Huntsman staff came to view Karen as an exceptional treatment responder. Starting in the spring of 2008, she saw Dr. Jensen on a quarterly basis, which meant a brain MRI on one day, followed by a face-to-face appointment with him a day or two later.

Sometimes, the suspense was simply too much, which is why I occasionally called the Huntsman even before the face-to-face appointment to ask one of my staff contacts the MRI scan results. Whatever the news, I would keep it to myself. If it were good news, I wanted to see the joy on Karen's face when she heard it from the doctor; if it were bad, I had lead-time to comfort her.

Because Dr. Jensen has been in the "brain" business for decades, it was particularly satisfying when he would announce that, once again, he saw no evidence of disease (NED) in Karen's brain from the most recent MRI scan. How did he know there were no tumors? What would he look for?

The beautiful thing about digital MRI scans is that they display results, in shades of black and white, on a computer screen in the exam room. As the room's lights came down, there was Karen's brain, and the longer we were on this journey, the more we knew what to look for. As Dr. Jensen rotated the brain view 360°, Karen and I could see her entire brain, including areas from past surgeries, radiation necrosis, and potential problem areas. These were powerful images, not a little bit unnerving. Our greatest concern was spotting those small, white-ish orbs that could appear anywhere in the brain, evidence of cancer growth.

To everyone's amazement, these quarterly appointments yielded the same incredible results: Karen's brain was "quiet" and normal. There were no glowing orbs or bleeding, dying, radiated tumors. When it was clear those were the scan result, smiles would break all around the exam room, as Karen had been given more time to live and thrive. Truly, those were memorable appointments, some of the happiest times for us at the Huntsman.

Good news called for celebration, which meant that after the scan results appointment, Karen and I headed to the 6th floor's Pointe restaurant for a delicious meal; to repeat out loud again the news we had just heard and seen with our own eyes; to speculate on what was coming next; and to draw strength from the beauty just outside the restaurant's panoramic windows. Our Pointe meals together are some of the best memories I have with her.

Dr. Jensen directed Karen to continue taking Keppra, her anti-seizure medicine, until further notice. In generic form, it was a relatively inexpensive medication, with no noticeable side effects in Karen, and it served as "insurance," a way to make future seizures less likely. The good news was that after several more quarterly MRI's continued to show no-evidence-of-disease, Dr. Jensen stretched Karen's MRI scan schedule to every six months. Those were incredibly rich months; up to that point, Karen had dodged a death sentence.

Unfortunately, NED does not mean remission, that the cancer is gone. I so wish it did. Cancer lurks in dark corners. It is relentless and evil; the body's cells running wild. It does "head fakes," fooling even the most experienced physicians. Melanoma cancer, in particular, loves to metastasize to the brain, slowly impairing the bodily functions, personality, and memory of a human being. In spite of this tough enemy, Karen and the physicians were doing all they could do to fight the battle, and with the good news we were receiving from Dr. Jensen, our lives filled up with many joys.

Along with the periodic MRI's, Karen would either get a CT or PET (positron emission tomography) scan of her torso area at least every three months, to check the melanoma cell activity in that area. While cheaper, CT's could not track a tumor's metabolic activity, so PET's were used if the physicians could rationalize medical necessity to my insurance company. The theory was that the nursery for melanoma in Karen was probably in her right lung. Although her brain showed no new tumor activity, melanoma in her lung was still active. This activity was hard to extinguish; in fact, it never went away.

*****

In the spring of 2009, Karen's Wellness Center in-house strength and cardio training, and frequent outdoor bicycling, was in preparation for a life-altering event: participating in the women-only, Little Red Riding Hood (The Little Red) ride near Logan, Utah, the first Saturday in June. Started by a sixty-year-old woman over twenty years ago and staged in a large, open valley, the Little Red:
- Gave women a chance to ride bicycles
- In a non-competitive setting
- Covering between seventeen and one hundred miles
- Over a well-planned course
- With frequent, well supplied rest stops and lots of opportunities for socializing with women of all ages
- And minus the influence of male riders.

Karen had never done anything like this, but now, as a Stage IV cancer patient with a clear brain, she was game. Kim, her dear friend and Huntsman exercise specialist, was going to ride the entire thirty-five miles with her, a true lady's day out. Kim and Karen started training several months ahead of the event, and then The Ride Day, June 6, arrived.

Karen and I packed the car – her bike strapped to a roof rack – and left Sandy early morning for the 90-minute drive to Logan. As we drove north, other cars, filled with riders, joined us along the highway, and by the time we got to the starting point, we found the place packed with 2,500 female riders and their bikes. We met Kim at the Starting Line, took some pictures, checked tire pressures, and off they went.

Four hours later, Karen and Kim coasted triumphantly across the Finish Line, Karen's beaming smile telling me that it had been a fantastic experience. Of course, she had stories to tell, but even more importantly, a sense that she could do something extremely significant. Not only did she ride the entire 35 miles without incident and took home incredible memories, but she gained the respect of her co-riders. Celebrations followed at the Huntsman Cancer Hospital's special tent at the Finish Line honoring patients who were riding that day. Karen lingered in that space, soaking in the mood and the attention. She earned it, that's for sure.

To their credit, Little Red organizers had dedicated the entire Ride to raising funds for the Huntsman's cancer research, which meant that Karen was not only a rider, but, in the years ahead, a recipient of money given by the 2,500 women and their friends across the country for cancer research.

What an absolutely amazing day. I was never so proud of Karen, and like the Woman In The Bed experience, saw her in a new light. Why does it often take hardship and loss for us to see ourselves, our loved ones, and indeed life in general, in a different way? Some might "see" differently just based on reason; I had to face my own blindness by watching my wife strive to live fully, each day. Jesus said, "So do not worry about tomorrow; for tomorrow will care for itself. Each day has enough trouble of its own," (Matthew 6:34). Karen was all about this. I, too, was learning to live in the present.

*****

Riding in the Little Red clinched the deal. Karen was hooked on cycling, including riding in the spring Salt Lake City Bicycle Tour, which followed the route mapped out for the City's runner's marathon. Starting at 6 a.m., the non-competitive Bike Tour allowed riders to tear through the city without concern for stoplights or cars. Starting in 2010, Karen rode four years in a row, with friends from the Wellness Center, me one year, and in 2013, all by herself. Once at the Finish Line, she would join the other Wellness Center Hometown Heroes at the Huntsman's tent, to celebrate and swap stories. It was life giving.

Strange, but even in 2008/09, the reality of Karen's likely mortality caused by melanoma had still not sunk into me. I think the NED years, and her overall tenacity, like riding in the Little Red, faked us both out. On hindsight, I wish someone (maybe a social worker, or even one of our physicians) would have sat me down and said, "Sterling, Karen is likely terminal. Spend as much time as you possibly can with her. Build memories, share joy, and love. This no-evidence-of-disease intermission is a gift. Use it wisely."

Maybe they did say that, and I just didn't hear it.

On the other hand, I am not sure I would have understood the message even if I did hear it. We generally expect parents to die before us, certainly before our children. But in my case, when Karen got sick and was likely to die "before her time," well, emotionally at least, I could only handle so much "reality." The fact is Karen and I did a lot together while she had cancer, especially during those intermediate good years. Now, I would trade everything I own to have one more week with a healthy her.

I am not beating myself up about this, as I was doing the best I could.

So was she.

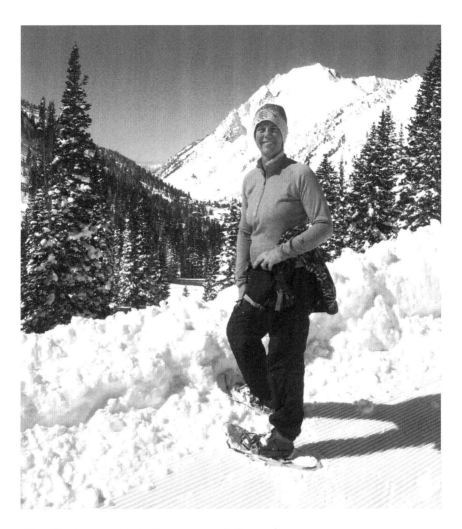

Alta Ski Area – Little Cottonwood Canyon

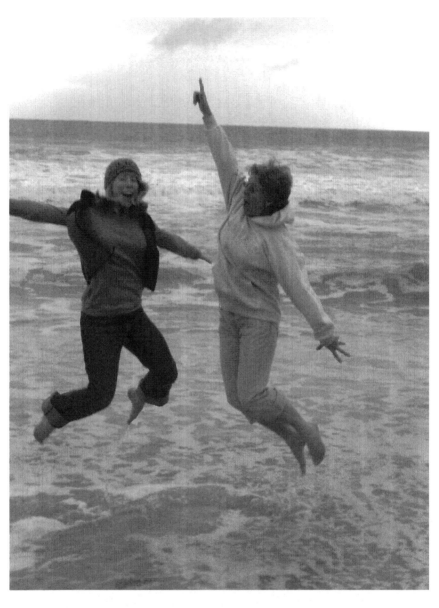

Allene, Karen – Oceanside, CA

~14~

Personality Changes

Who was Karen Swan? Ethnically, she was a mixture of Dutch and Swede, Dutch mostly.

The oldest of four children.

"Hard to handle," said her mother. "Always curious. Very athletic. Outdoorsy."

She was raised in a simple but comfortable home, where experiences, not things, were important to her.

Since Karen had a college degree in education, she homeschooled our four children for the first handful of their elementary years. She was a strong believer in "no child left inside," of getting kids out in nature and their hands dirty, and taking risks.

She was very social, with a large circle of female friends and a smaller, inner circle of kindred spirits, including one, Gail, who lived right across the street from us. Gail was one of the best friends Karen ever had, living out the meaning of love and trust.

Growing up in a small church in Southern California taught Karen the importance of service and gave her lots of opportunities to do so. Music and children were her special joy. She also participated in Bible Study Fellowship for many years. She loved cultures, geography, science – especially marine biology – and anything to do with the home.

She had trusted Christ as her savior at a young age, and as an adult, was a sincere follower of Jesus. Yet, she was no pushover. She had opinions and was never afraid to express them. Her parents had been missionaries in Guyana, South America, and before children, Karen and I traveled all over the world, including Central America, India, Israel, Europe, Canada, and the United States.

A practical person, Karen lived life for today; she would quickly say "yes," to an opportunity, and then follow through. As the idealist, I was often in awe at how she did this. As in any normal, long-term marriage, I learned a lot from her.

Filled with creative genes, Karen enjoyed sewing, cooking, gardening, drawing, home decorating, and playing violin and piano, among other things. She loved learning, and I still have hundreds of books scattered throughout the house to prove it. Animals were a vital part of her life; she loved all kinds, which explains why we always had at least one around the house (dog, cat, bird, etc.), often more.

All these friends, experiences, travel, hobbies and skills shaped Karen in profound, healthy ways. Clearly, though, apart from her marriage, the most importantly earthly gift to her was her four children. They were the joy of her life, and she threw herself into loving them in a way that any good mother does.

A month after Karen turned 49, things changed. With surgeries, radiation, medications (to fight melanoma and attempt to manage the side effects), Karen's personality evolved. How could it not? Her brain was continually traumatized, stressed, cut, heated, and drugged by very strong treatments, most only dimly understood by physicians.

In general, her personality, expressed in her interests, opinions, and activities, became more intense as the years progressed. Sometimes it was a challenge for me to keep up, but we worked at it, making it happen. On hindsight, it was probably better that Karen's biological response to the cancer and treatment was an intensified personality, as it helped her live life fully. The alternatives, such as physical impairment that trapped her at home, admission into a full-time care facility, or even her inability to drive a car ever again – were things we avoided.

Karen was driving a car again? Yes. Following her 2007 seizure, Dr. Jensen asked me not to let Karen drive until the brain calmed down. Once we started into the no-evidence-of-disease years, he said she could start driving again, and she did, often by herself, all the way through November 2013. This was important for us both. If she wanted to do something, off in the car she went.

If we were going through a tense relationship phase, she could head out to see a church friend, go to the Huntsman's Wellness Center, or horseback ride with Mim or a daughter. It was just who she was, who she had become. If I held back on participating in something, she would jump in the car and take off. "No opportunity left behind," was her motto.

Towards the end of the no-evidence-of-disease years, after we had been to the Huntsman for an infusion treatment, Karen and I left home to do some errands and I let her do the driving. We were literally just a block away from our home when she asked me for a scrap of paper so she could get rid of her chewing gum.

When I didn't respond quickly enough, she started rummaging around the car herself. Momentarily distracted, she took her eyes off the road, unknowingly turned the steering wheel right, and in a split second, half of the car was up on the sidewalk.

Rummaging around with her, I was also distracted. When I looked up, all I saw were three green, rectangular, four-foot high phone company boxes in my windshield. We plowed into two of them, mowing them down like corn stocks. I grabbed the steering wheel, turned it hard to the left, and yelled at Karen to stop, which saved us from hitting the third, larger box.

I was steaming mad, but Someone pulled me back from the edge.

Once we moved the car back to the house and our nerves calmed down, I thought about a few things:

- Accidents happen
- Those boxes were not telephone poles
- The high voltage going into those boxes did not electrocute us
- Our airbags did not deploy and we were uninjured
- My auto collision insurance reimbursed us for nearly the entire value of the car
- Our rates did not go up because it was a collision with an object, not another car
- Sandy police issued Karen a ticket for inattentive driving, which we paid
- Finally, she went to a one-night driving school, so the accident event was removed from her driving record

This accident illustrates that because of cancer, when it came to our relationship, there was never a dull moment. Karen was full-throttle engaged with life. Me? Trying to hold on. Most of the time I was able to adjust to these changes and, as the song says, "shake it off."

As I mentioned earlier, I decided that often saying "sorry" was a good thing, partly because I was making mistakes, and partly to placate Karen, trying to keep our lives from coming undone. Was this "apology behavior" genuine? Yes, mostly. It was my way of keeping peace in our relationship and family. It was a choice.

Saying sorry did not always work. Occasionally, we would have some serious, sustained fights. There was no hitting – ever – but certainly sharp disagreements. Even with the cancer, Karen was a very strong woman. One time, she kicked in a large chunk of wall near the kitchen with her foot. Just one blow took it out. Another time, she took her fist and drove it through drywall. No glove, just one powerful punch at shoulder height.

Both times, I was stunned. I never made any effort to repair either hole; she caused the damages, she could fix them. Months later, she did.

In another conflict, Karen and I disagreed over whether Neil should have a cell phone at his age or not. Seems rather petty, now, but in marriages, sometimes the small things become big things. When Neil told her I opposed the cell phone, she came rushing upstairs, stormed into our bedroom, and using her arm as a brush, swept all the items off the top of our six-foot long chest-of-drawers, including a camcorder, lamp, and treasured wooden box from India. Everything crumpled on the floor in a corner. Chaos ensued.

Karen won that battle; Neil soon got the cell phone.

*****

Karen had grown up learning respect for other people. Even with Stage IV cancer, she was normally still considerate. But when something spiked her impulses, all bets were off. For example, one day we drove to a local In-N-Out burger shop. As I pulled into a parking spot, another car pulled into the spot just to our right. The solo male occupant jumped out and ran into the restaurant, leaving his engine running and radio blaring.

That "music," rather innocuous really, suddenly agitated Karen. She jumped out of our car, opened the guy's driver side door, got in, and started trying to shut off the "noise." Unsuccessful, she tried to turn off the ignition.

In a panic, I pleaded with Karen to get out of the man's car. She would hear none of it. As I feared, the owner reappeared carrying a bag of burgers, to find my wife half way in his car.

She climbed out, got in his face, told him that the music was way too loud and annoying, and next time be more considerate.

To my great relief, the young man, probably in his 20's, calmly listened to Karen's complaint, apologized for the loud music, got in his car, turned off the music, and left. That drama over, the two of us went into In-N-Out, ordered our food, ate outside on one of the benches, and then went home. We had just dodged a bullet.

Fortunately, not every day was this intense. The reality, though, was that most days were a balancing act, an awkward dance where we frequently stepped on each other's toes. More than being "right," I was all about making sure she got her cancer treatments, a safe living situation, and every opportunity to live life to the fullest. Our evolving relationship strains were NOT Karen's "fault," or my "fault," rather, purely the nature of the beast. We were just human beings experiencing hardship and stress that was totally foreign to us, to our family, and friends.

Cancer sucks.

~15~

Children and God

Children need their mothers.

Karen was a particularly good one.

Our brains, still largely a mystery, host knowledge, skills, memories, experiences, personality and even spiritual reality, merged together in that way that is simply astonishing. Impact those cells – intentionally through trying to fight cancer, or unintentionally through a disease like dementia – and the "person," no matter how strong or determined, can potentially change.

In addition, in the case of cancer in the brain, there is the realization that bad things are going on in that person's control center, resulting in anticipatory grief: Karen could likely die "before her time." This is why my children faced challenges that few of their peers could even imagine, even as they sought to mature, make choices, find comfort, and engage with adult life. It was an immense test, a roller coaster ride with no seatbelts, for which there was no road map. It was a hand grenade thrown in the midst of our family, and when it exploded, the shrapnel penetrated each Swan in a different way.

I loved my children, but sometimes, especially in their younger years, I did not like them. I was distant. Detached. I say this with a great deal of sadness. Any rationalizations I might offer for this behavior are pathetically weak. In contrast, Karen, like most mothers, liked and loved her children. She gave them a wonderful gift of unconditional love and acceptance. I was learning to do this as part of my "Woman in The Bed" epiphany, the lessons coming most intensely after Karen died. After she passed away, I began to see each of my beloved children in a new light, something I will speak about towards the end of this book.

How did Karen's illness affect my children? Disorienting for some? Fostering spiritual disbelief? Anger? Sadness? Courage? Determination? Accelerated maturity? Even to this day, I am not sure. One thing is for certain; their lives will never be the same. As her illness stretched into the years, my children and extended family adjusted in a wide variety of ways.

My oldest son, Ryan, already out of the house except for some brief transition periods, threw himself into college, work, outdoor activities, and friends.

Amber graduated from Biola University in Southern California, and then moved back to Salt Lake to work and spend time with her mom. Later, she spent two years with AmeriCorps out-of-state during the no-evidence-of-disease years in Karen's brain.

Allene attended a local community college, transferred to Biola, and then decided to take some time off, coming back to Salt Lake to work and help out with Karen. She also joined AmeriCorps for two years, one year in Southern Utah, the other, Washington State.

While respectful of me, my relationship with my three older children waxed hot and cold. They were adults, launching out into life, learning lessons common for young people. In addition, learning to deal with their mother's chronic illness was a challenge far beyond the experiences of most of their peers.

Now in adulthood, each was relating to me in a new way, even as my relationship with their mother evolved. Karen was my primary focus; and while I knew that I was not connecting with Ryan, Amber, and Allene nearly as well as I would like, I simply did not know what to do, or have the energy to make it happen. The best we could do was what we did, place one foot in front of the other and press on.

Neil went through the teen years living with his ill mother, an experience that shaped him in profound ways for the rest of his life. My take on things is that he had to "grow up" quick. Like my three older children, he saw death first-hand, a defining moment in his young life.

Who takes a class on how to cope with anticipatory grief when it strikes? No one. Life simply happens; it goes on. Did we have family meetings, sitting around laughing, crying, sharing pains and joys? No. I think that would have been impossible. The "safest," probably most memorable things we did were in the outdoors: hikes, bicycling, horseback riding, and frequent trips to North County San Diego to enjoy the ocean.

*****

After the first intense year of Karen's illness, members of Karen's and my biological families responded to this long-term cancer marathon in rather predictable ways. My elderly mother lived in a Southern California retirement home and was not able to travel. One of my sisters, also in California, a widow with four children, had her hands full. My second sister was estranged from my biological family.

Karen's mother came up to stay with her several times while I continued my one-week-a-month contract job. In addition, her folks stepped in to help us financially during a particularly tough period early on. Karen's two sisters lived in California, and her brother lived and worked overseas. One sibling made it a point of regularly coming up our way. The others did not.

The 700 miles separating us from extended family meant that we were largely on our own. Occasional trips to Vista, CA made things a bit better. We certainly could have used more help, that's for sure. Should we have moved down to California? There were clear trade-offs. We would have gained some family support, but lost the Huntsman's holistic-care environment.

*****

Mothers often play the role of cheerleaders in their children's lives. In spite of the brain trauma, Karen did her best to stay engaged with her children: when they were in town, through lots of activities, especially outdoors; when they were away, primarily through phone calls, texts and photos. Texts were her favorite. It was an impressive sight watching her fingers fly over her phone's keypad, words coming together in a flash, texts going off into cyberspace, and then just as quickly, responses coming back.

My children's personality differences, geographical separation, work, school, and outside friends, meant that even traditional family events like Thanksgiving, Christmas and birthdays were hit and miss. There were some good times when we could all come together. There were also periods of time when simmering conflicts boiled over. I knew that part of that tension could be laid at my feet. Ours was probably typical family life issues, multiplied by the cancer dynamic, which meant that other forces were at work keeping us together.

Family issues aside, my children, especially Allene and Amber, regularly smothered Karen with love and attention. It was a sight to see, a marathon act of service, which deeply encouraged us both. Ryan, Karen's firstborn, was her pride and joy; when he was around, she lit up. I am sure that my three oldest children did more than I will ever know, tangible acts of love that probably kept me from a nervous breakdown.

Neil, six years younger than his sisters, responded to Karen's illness quite differently. While he stood on shifting sand at home, he found stability at school and church. Both environments provided solid adult and peer influences in his life and kept him moving forward. Reality was, though, Neil was just as human as his siblings, and although things seemed fine on the surface, there were some significant grief issues, stuffed while Karen was alive, that he began to address only after she died. Nonetheless, he regularly brought great joy into Karen's life during those long years, and like his brother and sisters, learned to serve in ways far beyond his peers.

As for me, well, among other things, this cancer journey was teaching me that I had been mad at God for extensive portions of my life. It was an unhealthy way to live; yet if Karen had not contracted cancer, I might have kept up the facade up for some time.

Dream on, Sterling! Her disease made the act unsustainable.

Problem was, I had acted so long that I could hardly wrap my arms around an authentic Faith. Over time, I became bitter, both at church and God, and I have little doubt that my children saw this bitterness and perhaps even copied it. For a while, I stopped regularly going to church. My choices were a terrible example to my children at a critical time in their lives, behavior and attitudes that I so regret now. I am so sorry. God is all about redemption in the midst of human frailty, truth that gives me hope for the future.

Complicating my spiritual confusion was jealously, as I saw other Christian families who appeared doing well. Life was clicking for them: their kids were hanging around good friends and getting married; they were diving into careers; the husband and wife were getting along; and Faith was important to them.

In contrast, my wife had terminal cancer, and my family was upended, tossed in the air. Was her cancer God's way of punishing me, like the Old Testament character, Job?

The Bible often speaks about how pride keeps us from truly knowing God. This was true for me. Karen's illness was the tool used to strip off my pride, one layer after another. Even though I was male, first-born, highly responsible, and a former air traffic controller, I was struggling to cope and deal with my loneliness.

Nevertheless, I was not alone. While this soul renovation hurt, I have come to realize that God was holding all six Swans in the palms of his hands.

Only it would take time for me to accept that he really cared.

~16~

Caring For Me

With the "responsibility gene" in my DNA, I did a good job taking care of the mechanics of Karen's illness (insurance, appointments, interactions with physicians and staff, etc.). I also needed strokes, affirmations from people to keep me from burning out. A number of things helped.

ARUP –
I regularly gave platelets at ARUP, which supplies all the blood products for four hospitals in the Salt Lake Valley, including the University and Huntsman Hospitals. Why would I do such a thing when my wife was in a cancer hospital? Although I had started donating years before Karen got sick, I continued because:
1) She used platelets, and it was a way for me to give back,
2) It was a place of solace, and
3) The staff there liked me, especially the older nurses who had known me for years. When they found out Karen had cancer, they always ask about her *and* me.
ARUP got my platelets; I got attention from some wonderful people.

Huntsman Cancer Hospital Volunteer –
For twelve months, starting in 2011, during some of Karen's no-evidence-of-disease (NED) years, I volunteered ten hours a week in the Huntsman's extensive outpatient clinics. My fellow volunteers and I had a specific assignment: Provide free snacks to the patients, family, and friends who were waiting in the five large outpatient clinics, and give a listening ear if they wanted to talk.
Often they did.
I was in my element. I loved interacting with folks from the multi-state region served by the Huntsman. In many ways, they were like refugees, fighting the battle of their lives, arriving on the Huntsman's doorstep shell-shocked. Not infrequently, we talked

for 10-15 minutes, sometimes longer, right there in the waiting areas. Others would often listen in. When they learned that Karen was a patient, too, the questions flowed. Over time, it was not uncommon to recognizing returning patients and their families, and often, they would spot me, calling me by name. Serving at the Huntsman during those months made me feel deeply valued and energized.

"The King's Speech." –

Can a feature-length Hollywood movie transform a person? This one did for me. I saw the King's Speech, about a 20th-century English king, in early 2012, and it had a huge impact on the way I thought about myself.

I had grown up with a lot of chaos at home, so the way we coped was to not talk about all the bad things that were happening, how we felt about them, or even that they happened at all. The result was I learned to lie, to others and myself. The King's Speech, about a stuttering national leader, became a metaphor for me. I also stuttered, not literally, but in telling the truth. As a young person, I had developed a hesitation to tell the truth, often because it was too painful, or I was afraid of the consequences. This bad habit impaired me, affecting me all my life. I was weary of the results.

In the midst of Karen's illness, just as she was about to enter some hard years that would ultimately lead to her death, this movie was a lighting bolt, a reality check on how I wanted to deal with myself, others, and life. I realized there was power in telling the truth to others and myself. Truth was freeing. Why not begin thinking and speaking it going forward? Learning to tell the truth helped me care for myself.

Bicycle Riding –

I had grown up riding bicycles all over my hometown area of Torrance, California, continued it when I moved to the San Fernando Valley in the 70's and kept on pumping the peddles when we moved to Utah in 1984. Karen's cancer did not stop me; cycling for me was easy, free, physical, and an escape from all the medical intensity. Feeling the wind against my face served to clear out my head; pumping the pedals helped me control my high blood pressure.

Karen's growing love of cycling – she was strong, fast, and persistent – meant that we often rode together, either puttering around the neighborhood, grabbing some ten-mile runs, or even strapping bikes on our car's roof and heading out to a designated bike path for the day.

I loved riding, by myself or with Karen. Today, her bike hangs from the ceiling in my garage. One of my daughters rode it in the June 2015 Little Red Riding Hood event.

Do I still ride? Yes, although after a recent crash, it's time for a new model. I am ready to hit the road again.

A Good Friend –

I had many acquaintances in the Salt Lake Valley, and a handful of good friends. After Karen got sick, my circle of friends began to shrink. Often this happens as men get older, but I could have used more friends, not less.

Fortunately, I had Rod. He and I met in Southern California during the late 70's, developed a strong friendship there, which continued even after Karen and I moved to Salt Lake City in 1984. Rod, a small business owner, highly relational and a sincere Christian, loved my family and I. His actions showed it.

When my caregiver stress – medical issues, relationships with Karen, the children or extended family, or my desperation – was about to take me over a cliff, I would go on a walk to a wilderness area near my home, call Rod, and unload.

He was a great listener; still is. Due to the nature of Karen's illness and how it was affecting our relationship, there was not a lot he could do to "solve" things, but solutions were really not what I needed. Rather, I just needed a non-judgmental friend who would allow me to go crazy, rant, whine, complain, scream, and then, tell me "this, too, shall pass. I'm praying for you, Ster."

There were periods when I would not call Rod at all, and then other periods when I would call him day after day. If Rod were busy when I called, he would always call back. Always.

There were some very dark days during Karen's long cancer journey. I remember one period where I was so close to giving up that I decided that I wasn't going to call Rod anymore, or respond to his calls. I was done, burned out, horribly depressed.

After a few days, Rod guessed that I was seriously depressed. He started calling me daily, and if I did not answer, left messages, which I randomly listened to, reminding me that he was there for me, that we were "brothers," and that I should not ignore him.

His persistence eventually helped me climb out of a deep hole. I started taking his calls once again, and eventually, calling him myself. No question, Rod was a Godsend. He is to this day, as we still talk a couple of times a week. This is what friendship is all about.

Coffee Guys –

Right after Karen got sick in the fall of 2006, I called a couple close Salt Lake friends from church and said, "I need you. Would you consider helping me keep my sanity through this tough time? Consider allowing me to call you on the spur of the moment so we could meet for coffee within a day or two. Think about this request and get back to me."

Both guys signed up. If one were busy, I would call the other one. We would meet early in the morning and spend about an hour together. There is no doubt that these two Christian men helped me from going over the edge. It's too bad I had not yet seen The King's Speech movie yet, as I was still holding back from them parts of who I was. No matter. They cared for me. One of the men was also my go-to person for shuttling Neil back and forth from school if I was with Karen at the Huntsman and could not pick him up myself.

I met with one of these men at least weekly for over the first two years of Karen's illness. Once she got to the no-evidence-of-disease phase, the need lessened and the three of us went on to other things. Nevertheless, those months together were some of the best memories I have during the seven years of Karen's illness.

A psychologist –

Did I seek out any kind of counseling during the years Karen was sick? Yes, several types.

Although not a marriage counselor, John Conley, the Huntsman social worker helping us navigate the cancer road, would meet with me if Karen and I were going through a crisis. He never said no, but I also knew that wasn't his job. Longer term, I looked other places.

Other places included a counselor I got through a referral, who seemed to have more needs than I had. I "fired" him after one session.

I was initially more hopeful about a second counselor, a man with a doctorate in psychology, lots of clinical experience, from my Faith tradition, and covered by my insurance. He and I met irregularly for over a year.

Unfortunately, I had not yet confronted the habitual dishonesty about how I was thinking and feeling. Result? The counseling sessions were largely a waste of time, energy, and money. In addition, the counselor had never gone through the type of hardship I was facing, so his approach with me missed the mark. Over time, our relationship strained, so much so that I started using absurd humor to express my displeasure.

In spite of this disconnect, he agreed to see Karen and I together a few times. Normally this is not done, but desperate times required desperate measures. Like my solo appointments, our sessions with him were largely unproductive; we would drive to the office not talking much, and leave not talking much.

On hindsight, it really wasn't the counselor's "fault." His efforts might have kept my marriage from completely blowing up, and because he was a Christian, I appreciated his prayers for me, even if I didn't really think God cared all that much at the time. It is more likely that the complexities of my marriage – Karen's brain impairment, my lying for so many years, and the brevity of the counseling sessions – made our situation very challenging even for the best of counselors.

I finally terminated the counseling towards the end of 2010; right around the time our trip down the turbulent cancer river would face new challenges and opportunities.

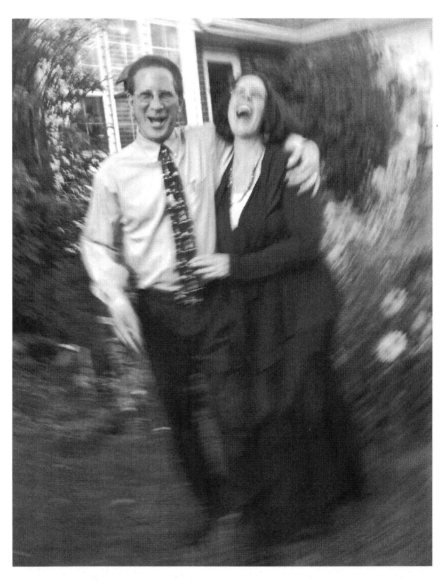

On our way to the Huntsman Cancer Foundation Gala

~17~

Clinical Trials

December 2010

The two years of no-evidence-of-disease in Karen's brain was an amazing run, allowing my family to build many good memories together, especially outdoors, in the mountains east of Salt Lake City, and on the beach just west of Vista, CA, where Karen grew up. While the cancer cells, surgeries, radiation, medications, and stress had affected her brain, she pressed on, as did our children and I.

During that period, Dr. Jensen, Karen's neurosurgeon, continued to see Karen every three to six months, carefully examining the periodic MRIs for any telltale signs of new melanoma orbs. Those were exciting days when, with a big smile, he would announce, "I see no new signs of tumors in your brain."

Unfortunately, Karen's cancer was far from gone. Periodic CT scans showed melanoma activity in her right lung, confirmed by more precise, expensive PET scan, which could measure cell metabolic levels. The result? Images on the exam room's computer displays were dramatic and worrisome.

To everyone's surprise, these melanoma cells were unusually restrained; they could have grown exponentially over the previous year, but did not. This passivity would not last. When campfire embers are deprived of fuel, or doused with water, they start to die down; yet these same embers can roar to life at a moment's notice if more fuel appears or wind picks up.

By the end of 2010, something in those melanoma cells started to fan tumor growth. In contrast to normal cells, melanoma cells consume the body's sugars at a voracious level; that is why they would show up bright yellow/white on a PET. In addition, a recent CT scan showed a new tumor, about 1cm in diameter, in Karen's left lung, also likely melanoma.

Gratefully, Karen had been in the eye of the cancer hurricane for almost two years, where the winds were relatively calm. Now, the winds were picking up. Trouble was brewing.

We continued to juggle seeing two oncologists, Dr. Akerley at the Huntsman, and Dr. Samlowski in Las Vegas. The stakes were simply too high to rely just on Dr. Akerley since his specialty was not melanoma. The two physicians collaborated via phone and email about Karen's care; when there was a professional difference of opinion, Karen always went with the one held by Dr. Samlowski. This did not threaten Dr. Akerley; even better, because of my PPO insurance, if Dr. Samlowski recommended a certain course of treatment, we could always get it at the Huntsman, all except for one procedure yet to come.

Towards the end of 2010, a new medicine became available, a potential game-changing approach to treating melanoma. Like Interleukin, which Karen had used four times in early 2007, it was designed to stimulate the patient's immune system; unlike that older drug, this new one was potentially more effective, and could be administered in an outpatient infusion setting. Its appearance on the scene was timely; we needed to douse the melanoma embers in Karen's lungs before they got out of control.

This drug was going through the FDA-mandated three-phase clinic trials. The Huntsman, one of the nation's national cancer centers, was a test site. What is a clinical trial? Before the FDA approves any drug for general use within the United States, the dosing, efficacy, and side effects are evaluated in people who have the disease or condition. This three-step trial sequence requires patients to volunteer to take drugs that might or might not help their condition, could greatly complicate their lives, or even cause death. Participating in a clinic trial was no small matter. Patients show tremendous courage when they volunteer, with no promise of a good outcome.

Karen was eligible for the third phase of the clinic trial testing Ipilimumab, (brand name: Yervoy), created by an American pharmaceutical company to specifically target melanoma. It was one of the first of many, many similar drugs now on the market, developed under a new treatment strategy called immunotherapy. The theory: provoke the body's own immune system to aggressively go after cancer cells.

Because this was a clinic trial, the medicine itself, delivered via four infusion visits in an outpatient setting, was free. Free was important, since once approved by the FDA, this drug would be priced at tens of thousands of dollars per dose retail. To participate, there was paperwork, lots of it. Karen read dozens of pages of trial documentation, initialed each page, signed the last one, and then witnesses added their signatures. In addition, throughout the trial, she would go through a battery of blood tests to monitor her organs' response to this medicine. This was serious, life-and-death business.

In short, Karen was at the right place at the right time; the chance to have a game-changing melanoma drug tested on her, at a wonderful facility only 30 minutes from our home, and all free. Her participation would also provide physicians, pharmaceutical and insurance companies, and the FDA, valuable information on the drug's efficacy and side effects. Consistent with her nature, she was all in.

"When can I start," she asked after Dr. Akerley pitched the opportunity?

"Immediately," was his response.

So it would be.

Once preliminary lab tests were complete, her first outpatient infusion appointment was scheduled at the Huntsman. Karen had already gone through four inpatient infusions; this was the first one in the outpatient setting, and on that appointment day, she was understandably nervous and a bit feisty.

*****

We arrived at the Huntsman infusion room lobby and checked in, only to have staff tell us that pharmacists were mixing the medicine, Ipilimumab (nicknamed: Ipi), requiring us to wait. This compound was so expensive that the hospital could not afford to have it just sitting on the shelf. Half an hour later, we got the green light; Karen's first dose of Ipi was ready.

I vividly remember what happened next. A medical assistant walked Karen into the Infusion Room, already filled with other patients, and led her to a vacant, solidly built recliner chair where she would sit while the drug dripped into her veins. Large windows looked east, towards beautiful snow-covered mountains, a view

Karen wanted to see, but couldn't, because the chair faced the opposite direction, towards a wall.

That wouldn't do! Flashing a mischievous smile, Karen grabbed that bulky recliner, spun it around with one quick move, and plopped down, victorious.

It was a dramatic entrance; she was her own woman. That was my Karen! I looked around the infusion room. Support staff and other patients were looking at Karen in amazement, as though collectively thinking, "I didn't know patients could do that. Is that allowed?" Karen wasn't asking; she just did it. A specially trained infusion nurse appeared, introduced herself, took one look at the chair's position, smiled and said, "You do whatever makes you comfortable." We were off to a good start.

Next, the nurse inserted an IV needle into one of Karen's veins and started a saline drip. She carefully read the contents of a tiny drip bag containing Ipi, read Karen's name out loud as she asked Karen to verify her name, and then called a colleague over to double-check all the information. That done, she added a special device in-line to the second drip tube, designed to make sure that every last milliliter, every last drop of Ipilimumab, made it into the infusion tube and ultimately into Karen's body.

Preparations complete, the nurse initiated the drug drip. I sat right next to Karen. We talked. Read. Looked out the large picture windows. She listened to her iPod and talked with staff and other patients. I ran to get some coffee. She crocheted. We ate snacks passed out by the staff, and together people watched, as patients came and went: old; young; vibrant; hurting; smiling; sad; male and female; alone, and those with caregivers, family, and friends.

Two hours later, the Ipi bag was empty. Time to head home.

How will a person respond to Ipilimumab and cope with side effects? It is a random wild card, based largely on an individual's biology. Fortunately, Karen's body handled this and three succeeding infusions, one a week, just fine, information that would be captured in great detail in the Clinical Trial database. She blew through all four doses, in four weeks, with nary a side effect. That, too, was my Karen, The Exceptional Responder.

In contrast, three years later, a close friend of ours, who also had Stage IV melanoma, attempted immunotherapy treatment using Ipilimumab. Even though he was physically fit and highly motivated, he was not able to complete even one dose, as the side effects were both immediate and severe. Ipi was not aspirin, that's for sure.

After four weeks and four doses of Ipilimumab, Karen was done with the Phase III clinic trial. Time would tell to what degree this medicine helped stimulated her immune system to kill, or at least slow the growth of the melanoma hot spots in both her lungs.

*****

With that treatment behind us, we drove to Las Vegas in March 2011 for another appointment with Dr. Samlowski. Her response to the four-dose infusion pleased him. He was less pleased with our answer to the next question: Had she received any radiation to the lung area following the four Ipilimumab doses?

No.

Dr. Samlowski leaned back in his chair, closed his eyes for a few moments, and then in his strongest tone to date said, "You should get radiation to that area as soon as possible."

Karen and I looked at each other, confused. Why radiation?

He explained that recent evidence showed that immunotherapy and radiation, done simultaneously, could create a compounding effect in attacking cancer, something akin to "the whole is greater than the sum of the parts" in some patients. And since Karen had her Ipilimumab infusion sequence about a month ago, the window for this compounding effect was closing.

A bigger bang for the treatment "buck?" Karen was all about this. Now, what to do?

While the Huntsman Cancer Hospital had just hired a new melanoma oncologist, we had yet to meet him. For a variety of reasons, we could not get the radiation that Dr. Samlowski recommended done at the Huntsman, so he gave us a referral to a former radiation oncologist colleague, currently practicing at another large cancer facility in the Salt Lake Valley.

Within a week we were in Dr. Watson's office, discussing the merits of conventional radiation (ten low-intensity treatments over a period of two weeks) to Karen's right lung, one stereotactic body radiation (SBRT) procedure to the tumor in her left lung, surgery, or both.

He believed traditional surgery in her left lung was too risky because of the tumor's location, recommending stereotactic radiation on the left side and conventional radiation on the right. Not one to over-analyze things, Karen said, "Make it happen. I want both."

Within a few days, Karen started conventional radiation. She was in and out of the radiation room in fifteen minutes.

Repeat ten times.

Then came the stereotactic body radiation (SBRT), a one-time procedure: Targeting was done and confirmed; the computers were programmed; radiation was generated; and that was that.

Mission accomplished.

Sort of...

*****

Karen's previous radiation treatments were all performed at the Huntsman, and as the bill-paying guy, I was familiar with their procedures. This new provider ran things differently, dramatically so. When I received the Explanation Of Benefits from Blue Cross, I was in for a shock. They had rejected the bill for the stereotactic body radiation charges, disputing the procedure's medical necessity. In their view, Karen should have received ten doses of low-power, conventional radiation to this left lung tumor, not the much more expensive stereotactic body radiotherapy.

Since I had never received an insurance denial for such an expensive claim in over four years, the appeals process was a brand new, steep learning curve. So began a yearlong battle for payment. I soon realized that there had been massive miscommunication between the hospital and myself regarding prior approval for the $14,000 stereotactic radiation treatment. What happened? Essentially, I expected they would follow steps similar to those used by the Huntsman when expensive procedures were needed. They did not. Now, in the hospital's opinion, I was on the hook for $14,000.

I told Karen nothing about this problem; she had other things to worry about. Worse case scenario, I would eventually have to pay the $14,000. Although I was a long way from throwing in the towel, I was also running out of appeal ideas. The hospital would not budge, and neither would Blue Cross when I contacted their Call Center. It was like a months-long tennis game between these two organizations, with the likelihood that the ball would eventually land in my lap.

Except it didn't.

As I re-read my insurance contract, looking for another angle in the appeals process, out jumped a paragraph about a patient advocate, a staff person with Regence Blue Cross who could potentially help me navigate the payment "corn maze" I found myself in.

I immediately made a phone call to Linda, a Regence employee and claims appeal specialist. While this SBRT situation was fairly complex, she assured me she would promptly "get to the bottom of things," reprocess the claim based on what I had told her over the phone, and equally important, advocate for Karen.

Several weeks passed. One day I got a call from Linda, immediately apologetic. An internal review had again denied the claim. Regence's medical department staff still viewed stereotactic body radiotherapy as elective and investigational.

*****

Stunned, I was at the point of giving up. One day, "out of the blue," an answer came to me, insight beyond myself or any other person I had spoken to. The insight: become a medical insurance contract expert!

I threw myself into reading and understanding Regence's medical policies, which are detailed, medically-specific guidelines undergirding every conceivable type of medical procedure, from removing a sliver to brain surgery. These medical policies discuss in detail subjects such as what the insurance company would pay, standard versus investigational care considerations, and what a physician would have to rationalize to get a cutting-edge procedure approved by the company. They are the foundation upon which a patient's medical plan is built.

Like the Wizard of Oz, using the Internet and Dr. Watson's detailed notes, I pulled back the "curtain" behind a patient's insurance coverage and taught myself to speak medical policy language. Once I had this figured out, I wrote Regence Blue Cross a lengthy letter, tying the doctor's detailed rationale for using the SBRT radiation procedure with his line-by-line written references to the Blue Cross medical policy, and included Regence's own web pages, policy links, and interpretations.

I felt like I was in court, making my case, presenting evidence and calling witnesses! Once done, I mailed all this documentation to Linda at Regence, who, seeing I had done my homework and believing I had a good case, took the proactive step of putting Karen's SBRT procedure out for external review. This last-chance analysis, by a respected physician who was not affiliated with the insurance company, allowed for a fresh look at her case.

Linda did not have to do this, but she did.

On May 11, 2012, the Friday before Mother's Day and over a year after Karen's left lung SBRT treatment, I received a call from Linda. Moving out to the front porch so Karen would not hear me, she said, "I wanted you to know that I just received the results from the external review of Karen's claim appeal. The physician stated that SBRT was the only wise choice for treating the tumor in Karen's left lung and that it was clearly a medical necessity.

"With that, I will be re-processing the claim immediately. Allowed charges for the radiation will reflect the contract discount we have with the provider. Regence will pay the vast majority of the contracted amount; your responsibility is a bit over $1,100. Please wish Karen a happy Mother's Day."

I was so relieved I started weeping while I was on the phone. Moments later, before we said our goodbyes, I asked Linda if she would call the hospital's billing office that day notifying them of this decision, since they had been regularly hounding me for payment. She promised she would.

Dr. Watson had been right all along; SBRT was the only way to treat that tumor.

People whom I had never met, in this case, Linda, working in an office several states away, and a physician, who looked at Karen's case with fresh eyes, unknowingly became agents of God as they diligently worked on Karen's and my behalf, seeking to do the right, ethical thing. Answered prayers, often ones I personally did not pray, allowing me to shed some financial stress and move to the next chapter of the journey.

Finally!

Right on the heals of this bill resolution, two friends drove up from California to spend a week with Karen and I, hanging out in the Salt Lake area for a couple days, and four in Yellowstone

National Park. We reserved rooms in the iconic Old Faithful Inn, before the wave of summertime tourists arrived and had the time of our lives. Words cannot express just how much this couple cared for us. It was one of the highlights of our long cancer journey, and a fantastic way to celebrate the recent great news from Regence Blue Cross.

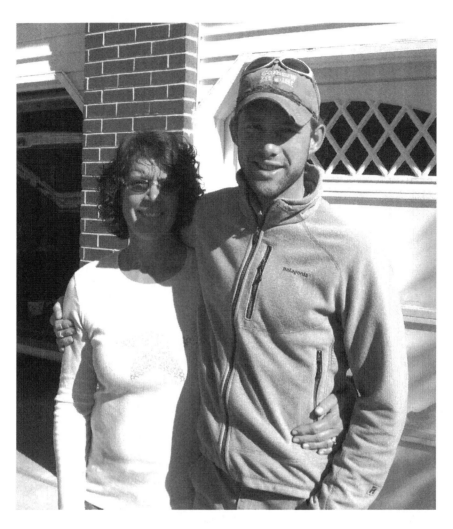

Karen, Ryan – Sandy, UT home

~18~

A New Oncologist

Just a few months after the resolution of Karen's lung radiation bill, Dr. Watson, the radiation oncologist that had provided the lung radiation treatments, took a job out-of-state. In cancer care, as in life in general, nothing ever remains the same.

Which is why Karen and I were grateful, not only for the Huntsman's proximity to our home, but the highly competent, specialized oncologists and support staff that worked there. Cancer care had become so complex that specialization, within one or two types of cancers, was the only way to fully serve the patients.

As a result, even though Dr. Akerley had provided Karen quality care, once spring 2011 arrived, she wanted to transition to Dr. Kenneth Grossmann, the Huntsman's newly hired melanoma oncologist. Drs. Samlowski and Grossmann knew each other well, the latter viewing the former as a mentor. They were professional, not territorial or competing, and their whole focus was on quality care for their patients, wherever that care could be obtained.

We knew they had a relationship of mutual respect just by the way they spoke about each other, creating a climate of trust that supported our use of their combined wisdom. This "pooling of the minds" certainly helped Karen, and took pressure off the oncologists to have every medical issue always figured out.

Without skipping a beat, Dr. Grossmann took the hand-off from Dr. Akerley as Karen's primary care oncologist at the Huntsman, while Dr. Samlowski continued serving as our trusted source of second opinions. Equally valuable, Karen and I both "clicked" with Dr. Grossmann's personality and love of science. He not only allowed time for "science-type" cancer questions during appointments, he invited them, which won us over.

In spite of Karen's recent success with the four-dose treatment of Ipilimumab and radiation to both her lungs, new CT and PET scans mid-spring 2012 showed good news/bad news. The good news was that the SBRT radiation had scored a bulls-eye on the tumor in her left lung, and that area now appeared "cold." The bad news? Karen's right lung, which some thought might have been the original source of the melanoma, was still hot.

Were those hot spots necrosis (dying tissue) from the surgery or recent radiation, swelling from either, or something else? Perhaps there were new tumors in the area, slowly starting to grow? Confirmation would come via a needle biopsy, entering Karen's lung through her back.

At the University Hospital, specialists perform biopsies on difficult parts of the human body. From an outsider's perspective, the idea of a needle going into a lung to grab a piece of tissue might seem dramatic, but after so many "dramatic" events, we viewed this procedure as rather routine. In Karen's case, a specialist extracted a small piece of lung tissue from the area in question, and the biopsy that followed showed non-malignant cells. That was outstanding news.

Dr. Grossmann gave us more good news. While Ipilimumab pressed Karen's immune system to go after melanoma cells, a parallel research effort had determined that certain genes controlled very specific functions within the body. In the case of melanoma, about half of all people have changes (mutations) in the BRAF gene. These changes cause the gene to make an altered BRAF protein that signals the melanoma cells to grow and divide quickly. Some new drugs, undergoing clinical trials, target this and related proteins.

In brief, the treatment concept was to use a chemical (in the form of a pill) to turn off this BRAF gene, which would perhaps stop the melanoma cells from growing and dividing. This thesis, like many other novel cancer treatment approaches, offered hope, but was it correct? Although the Huntsman did not have a clinical trial in this area, one of Dr. Grossmann's colleagues in Southern California did, so Karen and I set up an appointment, made the drive to West L.A., and met with the research oncologist who was running the study for a pharmaceutical company.

Although Karen was technically eligible for the trial, several things shot it down:
- There was no personal chemistry between her and the oncologist.

- Treatment would require frequent travel to the Southern California clinic for extended periods of time.
- Side effects could be horrible, especially for someone who loved the outdoors, including severe sunburns to any part of skin exposed to the sun after as little as 15 minutes.

Ultimately, any one of these was a showstopper. Karen got all the way to the last page of the clinical trial consent document, stopped, thought, put down her pen, and said, "NO!"

Although a bit startled, the clinical trial coordinator wished us well and we were out of there, hopping on the 405/5 freeways to see friends in Bakersfield. Two full years would pass before Karen reconsidered using any BRAF-inhibitor drugs.

*****

By the time we got back in to see Dr. Grossmann, he had heard from his colleague in Southern California. Admittedly, it did not go the way any of us had expected, but at least we tried. In the meantime, Ipilimumab had gone all the way through the FDA approval process and, rumor had it, would become available for widespread use literally any day. According to FDA rules, Karen was eligible for one more round of four doses, and since she breezed through the last round in January, Dr. Grossmann recommended she consider another treatment.

What was her answer?

"Yes, absolutely! When can I get it?"

FDA approval of Ipi was so recent that Karen was the first Huntsman patient to use this drug in the post-trial environment, which meant staff behind-the-scenes went to work acquiring the drug from the pharmaceutical company. As this occurred, Dr. Grossmann was drafting a letter to my insurance company justifying his decision to use Ipilimumab in Karen for a second time, so they would (hopefully) cover the medication's cost. It was part of an oncologist's job that few non-patients see.

He did it well. Linda, with Blue Cross, again expedited the approval process, and with that written document in hand, Huntsman staff ordered the precious liquid from the pharmaceutical company, an order that was probably delivered to the Huntsman by armored car!

Drug research and clinical trials are extremely expensive, and since we live in a capitalistic country, the pharmaceutical company seeks profit, which partially explains why each dose of Ipilimumab was priced at tens of thousands of dollars retail. A course of treatment was four doses over four weeks. Retail price is not what Regence ultimately paid HCH, and HCH the pharmaceutical company, since there are contractual discounts which help drive the cost down; but still, every drop of Ipi counted, in more ways than one.

On infusion days, we now had the routine down pat. Like our last infusion experience, Karen turned the recliner chair around, this time to watch mountain bikers and joggers out the windows enjoying warm July weather. Once the precious Ipi started through her veins, we passed the time by reading, talking, eating, and people watching.

Four weeks later, Karen had successfully completed Round 2 of Ipilimumab, again with no side effects. Stunning! Huntsman staff was very pleased. So were we. Karen and I were quite aware that the FDA's approval timing, and Blue Cross's full payment of the Ipilimumab charges, was not steps we could have scripted. Other forces were at work, as they had been from Day 1, starting way back in the fall of 2006.

That was the end of Ipi for Karen.

In 2011, FDA guidelines only allowed two rounds of four doses each. If the melanoma "embers" in her lungs flared up again, other treatment strategies would be needed.

Granted a reprieve, her lungs stable and no evidence of disease in her brain, Karen threw herself into celebrating life for the next sixteen months. Live we did, mostly outdoors. Each day was a gift, including the first weekend in June 2012, when Karen, Allene, and Amber rode fifty miles together in the all-female Little Red Riding Hood non-competitive event.

50 miles, by a Stage IV cancer patient and her daughters!

Simply amazing.

Once again staged in the expansive agricultural Cache Valley northeast of Salt Lake City, the Little Red regularly sold out a few hours after registration opened. Karen's Huntsman Wellness Center connections allowed her to get three slots for the Swan women. To this day, Allene and Amber look back on that Friday/Saturday weekend – those hours spent with their mom, socializing with other women, and riding their bikes – with deep, lasting memories that will never leave them.

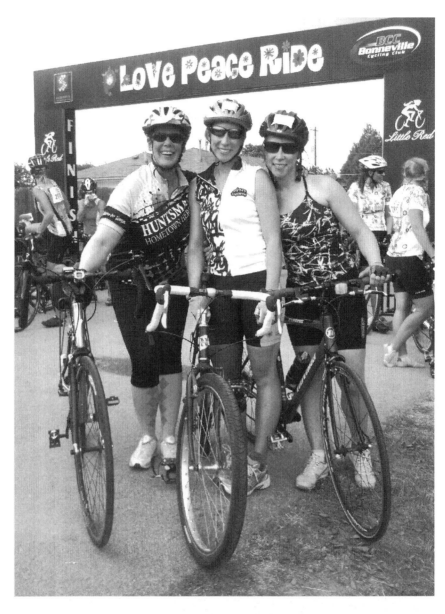

Karen, Amber, Allene – Little Red Riding Hood 2012 – Finish Line

~19~

Melanoma On the March

Those sixteen months of reprieve flew by.

We were shocked back to harsh reality in late 2012. Gathering with Dr. Jensen in an exam room to view recent MRI scan results, it was immediately clear that melanoma was on the march again in Karen's brain. New tumors, those hideous glowing white orbs, most about the size of pencil erasers, were clearly visible as Dr. Jensen rotated the 3D image around on the computer monitor.

Disappointment filled the room. Once that dissipated, we jumped back into the battle full force. New challenges were ahead; we would learn about them in due time.

Unlike Karen's first, tangerine-size tumor way back in 2006, these 5 to 10 millimeter-size spherical tumors were prime candidates for stereotactic radiation versus surgery. Dr. Jensen referred us back to Dr. Shrieve, the radiation oncologist who had treated Karen in 2006/07, with the expectation that she would likely undergo SRS soon, certainly before these tumors grew much larger.

*****

Fast-forward a few weeks.

When it comes to Stage IV brain metastasize patients, six years is a very long time. Unless he had kept track of her status the past years by periodically looking at her chart, for all Dr. Shrieve knew, Karen had died. Yet, there she was, sitting with me in an exam room in the Huntsman's outpatient radiation department.

A physician would never walk into a room and say, "Oh, I am shocked to see you are still alive." Yet to me, Dr. Shrieve 's body language said he was surprised and pleased, entering the exam room with a big smile and attentive manner. Karen *was* an inspiring survivor.

Longevity aside, the cancer beast was growing again in her brain. Dr. Shrieve and a fellow had already looked at Karen's most recent MRI scan done yesterday; once in the exam room, the images were displayed again so we could together discuss what they saw.

There were three tumors scattered around her brain, all slightly larger than when we had seen with Dr. Jensen a few weeks ago. Spherical and still relatively small, they were ideal candidates for stereotactic radiosurgery (SRS), which was far less invasive than surgery.

What about whole brain radiation? Dr. Grossmann, Karen's melanoma oncologist, was strongly against whole brain radiation treatment other than in dire circumstances. Dr. Shrieve agreed. Why? Whole brain treatment would likely involve a level of memory loss and compromise Karen's personality. SRS was the "safer" route and that was his recommendation.

Characteristically, Karen said, "Let's go for it."

What about the dreaded halo? That piece of metal was brutal.

Finally, Karen caught a break. In the years since her last SRS procedure, radiation medical technology had advanced; the dreaded halo was out, a "plastic-like," custom-made molded mask was in. Cause for celebration? Yes and no. Yes, Karen no longer had to endure screws twisted into her skull. No, the mask fit completely around her head, with spaces engineered for her eyes, mouth, ears, and airflow around her skull.

So the mask would make things a bit easier for Karen, on the continuum of do you want yourself poked with a hot branding iron, or a very hot branding iron? The new challenge was psychological, managing the claustrophobia and anxiety created by wearing this tight mask. In addition, Dr. Shrieve reminded us that while these tumor cells would be relatively easy to target due to their spherical shape, melanoma cancer does not go quietly into the night.

When hit with the radiation beam, the tumors tend to explode, rather than implode, causing residual bleeding in the dying tumor and scattering cancer cells in the immediate area. These common radiation results, plus swelling inherent in heating up the brain, meant that Karen would take steroids to help reduce swelling, ideally accelerating recovery.

Oh, great. Steroids again!

We had no choice.

This time around, it seemed like the psychological aspects of Karen's cancer battle increased dramatically. The no-evidence-of-disease years had given her a respite from this potential brain trauma; now it was back. In addition, her tolerance for any scan that involved sliding her head into a confined tube, or an object placed around her face, had declined.

For example, a preliminary SRS step called for Huntsman staff to put a mold around Karen's entire head, and from that, create a mask. Approaching this like "old times" five years ago, she went into the molding procedure with just her self-control. As the mold dried, all was going well until suddenly Karen reached up and started ripping everything off her face. Staff tried to convince her to relax, since the mold process was almost over, but anxiety had overtaken her. The damage was done; the mold ruined.

That was that.

Some days later, she came back for a second try, this time sedated with Valium. It helped. All went well. Staff got a good mask mold and went about crafting it for the upcoming SRS procedure. From that point on, I gave Karen either Ativan, or if the procedure was particularly intense, Valium, both anti-anxiety drugs, a half-hour before any procedure or scan.

*****

Towards the end of 2012, prior approval from Blue Cross in hand, targeting MRI brain scan complete, and computer programming finalized by Drs. Shrieve and Jensen, Karen lay on a Huntsman radiation table. Her head was restrained with the mask screwed into the table, her body held with straps, her music selections played on speakers in the radiation room, and Ativan, plus the prayers of many, calmed her psyche. Within minutes, radiation technicians would run the computer that would radiate three tumors – two about 5mm in size, one 10mm – all in one procedure.

A half hour later, it was over.

I met Karen in the dressing room, helped her change into street cloths, and then we had a short "going home" briefing from one of the nurses. Key instruction: Karen should take her steroids, full-strength at first, and then taper the dosage over the next few weeks.

As we knew from past SRS treatments, Karen and steroids did not get along, causing sleep loss, behavioral changes like agitation and impatience, and impulsiveness. But without the steroids, brain swelling and resultant headaches, or worse, were likely. Modern medicine had worked to save Karen's life to this point, but there were no easy solutions to complex biological challenges inside the confined space that was her brain.

Like past SRS treatments, the plan was to let Karen's brain settle down for a month or so, and then scan the area in January 2013 to see how things looked. Because of this, our family's 2012 Thanksgiving and Christmas holidays were quite subdued. That was fine. A highlight was Thanksgiving. My entire family was present as we shared a classic, home cooked turkey meal with all the fixings, creatively prepared by Karen and my daughters. Little did we know that life would be quite different in a year.

Black Friday, Internet Monday and free shipping from most retailers on the planet had no influence on us. Sometimes it felt like we were on another planet. As December rolled around, while steroid symptoms were showing their predictable face once again, Karen pushed through the tapering process and, eventually, was off that medicine. Christmas Eve came; again, everyone was there. After our traditional family meal of finger foods, five of us went to a local church for one of their services.

I recall the evening well. It was a cold December night outside, but warm inside the church building, a mood created by the people, music and decorations, and the many reminders of God's great gift in Christ. One of my favorite photos of this entire cancer journey was taken in the church's lobby that night. There we were, the five of us bundled up about ready to head out into the cold, standing close to each other with smiles on our faces, clearly happy to be together.

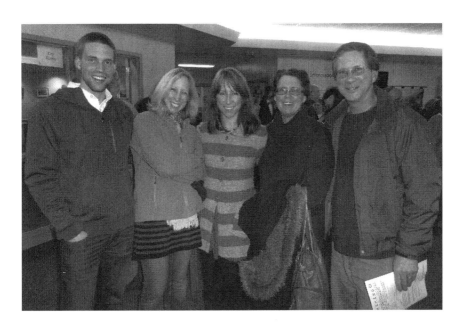

Christmas Eve 2012 – Neil, Amber, Allene, Karen, Sterling

~20~

Good News, Bad News

As 2013 arrived, Karen started experiencing symptoms that we had not seen before, primarily increased pain on the left side of her brain above her ear, occasional stability problems, and lots of fatigue. Fortunately, a follow-up MRI and appointment with Dr. Jensen we had previous scheduled for January came at a timely moment.

Unlike wiping a chalkboard with an eraser, radiating tumors using SRS does not always make bad things better; it sometimes only slows down melanoma's advance. As Karen and I gathering around the exam room's computer screen, Dr. Jensen explained that a couple of the tumors radiated last November appeared dead, while one, above her ear in the left temporal lobe, was bleeding. That bleeding was causing swelling and contaminating some of the other nearby brain tissue, increasing neurological side effects like irritability and sleep loss.

Why do some melanoma tumors explode, and others, not? Was it tumor age or size, intensity of the beam, or proximity to surgery? Drs. Jensen and Shrieve had done a statistical analysis of the hundreds of melanoma brain tumors they had radiated over the years, but found no clear patterns or explanations. For reasons yet unknown, these tumors just did as they pleased; some died a quiet death, while others exploded, bled, or both.

What to do with this bleeding? Although the topic was deadly serious, the setting for our discussion was relaxed. Karen and I sat together in one of the Huntsman's the two-person couches, Dr. Jensen grabbed the exam chair in the center of the room, and Melody, his ever-present nurse, stood over in a corner, taking notes.

As he saw it, there were three options: surgery to extract the obvious necrosis (dead cells from the radiation) and drain out the fluid; introduce more steroids; watch and wait, as sometimes the bleeding stops on its own and the body reabsorbs the blood. We kicked around the trade-offs of the three options, and then closing his eyes, Dr. Jensen leaned back slightly in the exam chair to think. The room went quiet.

Within a few seconds, he was back. "I would rather not do any more surgery," he said. "In 2006, I removed most of your right temporal lobe. Since then, the left one has carried the load. If I go in and remove part of that lobe, we don't know how it will affect you neurologically."

This was a stunning statement. Karen was absolutely not interested in a treatment option that could affect her personality or bodily functions. Neither was I.

"I want to watch and wait," she said.

So it would be.

Waiting and praying for Karen's brain to settle down gave us time to schedule appointments with Drs. Grossmann and Samlowski. Her last lung scans showed calm; now it was time for an update. We guessed that things had changed.

Late winter, early spring 2013 saw us heading to the Huntsman a lot, for scans, appointments, and the in-house Wellness Center activities. Fortunately, Karen caught several medical breaks:

1) While a PET scan showed activity in her right lung, it was not glowing hot. This news also bought us some time, since Dr. Grossmann and his colleagues were running out of bullets to keep those lung tumors at bay.

2) The follow-up MRI/visit with Dr. Jensen showed that the blood flow in her left temporal lobe, above her ear, had stopped and the radiated tumor was shrinking – leaving only necrosis, or dead cells – which meant that, at least for now, there was no need for surgery; and,

3) To Dr. Jensen's continual amazement, there was no evidence of tumor activity in or around the 2006 tumor surgery cavity above Karen's right temporal lobe, as if the tumor cells were miraculously all eliminated. Statistically, this was extraordinary.

*****

Unfortunately, it was too early to break out the wine. The most recent follow-up MRI showed several new melanoma tumors, one about 5 mm, the other, double the size, nearly 1 cm, in Karen's left frontal lobe (above her left eye).

Sobering.

Disheartening.

Exhausting.

Melanoma, the tenacious, insidious foe, was playing a deadly game of Whack-A-Mole with my wife.

Presented with the options – surgery or radiation – Karen went with SRS. Drs. Jensen and Shrieve concurred, as she had responded well to previous targeted radiation, was in overall good health, and Blue Cross would likely approve the treatment.

Karen was all in.

By now, the radiation routine was eerily familiar: Blue Cross prior approval in hand; targeting MRI, with Karen wearing the mask; physicians program the computer using complex 3D physics; procedure day – in and out; and going home, with instructions to use the steroids, high dosage at first, then taper in the weeks ahead.

*****

In mid-April 2013, Karen came back for another CT scan and appointment with Dr. Grossmann, where, sadly, we learned that the season of catching breaks was over. There was a new tumor hot spot in Karen's right lung.

We discussed possible options, including her joining a clinical trial there at the Huntsman, using a medicine that she had previously rejected because of reported harsh side effects. Now, with this lung tumor growth, the game had changed.

Whether to join the trial or not was academic, at least at this point, as we had to wait at least a month while Karen's brain calmed down from the most recent SRS treatment to her left frontal lobe. "Stabilize the brain," was still the prime directive; we would return to the Huntsman in a few weeks for another brain MRI to see how things looked.

Much was now outside ours, and the physicians', control. Karen's biology and her numbered days were driving events now.

~21~

"How Did You Do That?"

It was a raining on Friday night, April 19, 2013.

Exhausted, maybe this weather was the excuse I needed to bail out of the Salt Lake City Marathon ride with Karen the next morning? I secretly hoped she would bail, too.

What was going on with me? Didn't we have a good time last year riding the Marathon route together? What about all my talk about doing things with her as much as I could? I had paid the fee, so why not just go?

Ten hours before we were to leave for the Starting Line, I was in a funk.

Karen? Not a bit.

I even tried to talk her out of it. She would not budge; she was fully committed.

"If you are not going," she told me, "I will go by myself."

This was no bluff. She was going, for herself, and the companionship she enjoyed with other Wellness Center cancer patients riding the route (they were known as the Hometown Heroes).

We slept in separate beds for the previous few months, since I was snoring more and more and it drove Karen nuts, especially with her heightened sound sensitivity. The SLC Marathon Ride started at 6 a.m., at a pedestrian bridge on the University of Utah campus not far from the Huntsman Hospital, which meant we would need to get up at four in the morning, dress, eat, load the bikes into the car, drive downtown, get out the bikes, and get the start point, all before 6 a.m.

In the rain.

And cold.

Right before we both went to bed, I tried one last time to talk her out of going, using my last rational argument, essentially, "Since you just had brain stereotactic radiosurgery, shouldn't you reduce stress and avoid the risk of infection from a cold?"

Strong words went back and forth.
She would hear none of it.
She was going.

*****

I slept poorly that night, finally falling asleep around midnight. When 4 a.m. rolled around, I vaguely heard an alarm go off, movement in the master bedroom, kitchen noise, and then the garage door open. Before I knew it, the garage door closed.

Partly out of guilt, partly in panic, I rushed to the garage, only to see that the car was gone.

Karen was on her way.

Of the thousands of people who do this SLC Marathon Bike Ride every year, my guess is only a few have Stage IV tumors (of any sort) in the brain, much less just finishing a harsh radiation procedure one month earlier. This was the fifth time Karen had done this non-competitive ride. In years past, she had ridden with others from the HCH's Wellness Center, mostly with Patrick, her beloved trainer/coach/friend. Together, they would snake through the Salt Lake Valley, and by the time they reached the Finish Line, the odometer read 26 miles.

Karen told me later that on this rainy Saturday morning, she rode by herself, no Huntsman exercise specialist watching over her or buddies to help push her along. Fortunately, as in past years, the ride went normal; no falls or tire blowouts, etc. She told me she found it invigorating. She did see a couple people she knew on the road, including Patrick, but he was busy shadowing more needy patients, so she pushed on, swept along by the hundreds of others riders of all ability levels.

Crossing the Finish Line in downtown Salt Lake City, Karen immediately headed for the Huntsman Cancer Hospital's Hometown Heroes tent to grab some food and celebrate with "the gang." Patrick was already there, and he told me later that he thought he was seeing a ghost.

"How did you do that," he asked Karen, and by "that," he meant ride 26 miles, in the rain, by herself, and only a month after an SRS procedure on multiple tumors in her brain? Even though Patrick had known Karen, The Extraordinary Patient, for years, this astonishing effort blew his mind.

Yes, indeed, how <u>did</u> she do it?

She told me later that she socialized a bit with some of the other Huntsman riders in the Hometown Heroes tent. That was always a happy time for everyone. Equally impressive, when she was done, she took the city's light rail train back the Starting Point, disassembled her bike, put it in the car, and drove home.

Once home, Karen added the 2013 Ride completion medal to the other four that were hanging on a peg in our bedroom wall. Five rides in a row!

It was her last Marathon Ride.

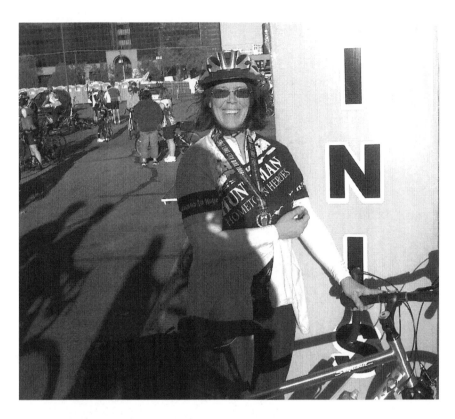

Salt Lake Marathon Bike Ride 2013 – Finish Line

~22~

Perseverating

A week after the Marathon Ride, Karen and I were in an exam room at our second home, the Huntsman, with Dr. Jensen. Gathered around the computer screen, all of us immediately saw the bad news: the recently radiated 1cm tumor in her left frontal lobe, above her left eye, was bleeding.

What to do? Recent history suggested that over time, the blood flow might stop, and then the brain, that amazing organ, would absorb the excess fluid. Since that was the outcome with her left temporal lobe, why not again? Karen chose "watch-and-wait" for a few weeks.

Dr. Jensen left the exam room to see another patient and his nurse said she would be right back, which left Karen and I alone. We looked at each other, our faces expressing a range of emotion that words could never begin to capture. I also thought out loud about her recent bike ride. As in so many other ways, so many other times, Someone was protecting my wife as she sped down Salt Lake City's streets in the early morning hours just one week ago, pedaling her heart out, solo, savoring the joy of the experience, even as a tumor bled in her brain.

The watch-and-wait plan meant several things, including a stop at Walgreen's on our way home to pick up our favorite medicine: steroids. Karen was absolutely fed up with steroids, and I didn't blame her, but I still convinced her at least to start. While we knew it was a strong dose, and the side effects that would likely follow, what alternative did we have?

*****

"Do you like gardening?"

"No!"

"Is Yama our cat?"

"No!"

"Do you want to go see Mim's horses?"

"No!"

Starting in early May, Karen's behavior, judgment, and information processing went off a cliff, plunging to a level of impairment that I had never seen before. Over just a few days, her adult vocabulary shrank to a dozen, childlike words, and the most common, No!

Worse, Karen was not even aware of what was happening, because her cognition had also been impaired. Adding to these complications, she would get agitated at the smallest thing, either around the house or with something I did or did not do. Increasingly, I was overwhelmed trying to get Karen to take her meds, including the steroids, along with eat, sleep, cooperate, and not hurt herself or damage the house. With each day, the crisis grew.

What about Neil? Couldn't he help? When he was at school, it was just me verses Karen, one-on-one. It felt like five-on-one. Even when he was home, I hesitated to saddle my teen son with stressful adult responsibilities involving his mom. He had already been through enough the last six years. In the couple times I did ask him to keep an eye on her while I ran out for food, upon my return, one look at his body language and face told me things had not gone well. That was way too much burden on him.

Desperate, I called Melody, Dr. Jensen's nurse. She suggested we try to stop the blood flow by increasing the steroid dose. Oh, great. More steroids. We might as well get in our car and drive off a mountain road together.

I gave Melody's suggestion a try, forcing Karen to swallow a larger dose.

Two days later, I admitted defeat; time for another idea.

Even more desperate, I again called Melody, explaining that things were coming apart at home. She responded by working us into Dr. Jensen's schedule two days down the road. It was the absolute best she could do, and I believed her. Counting the hours and biding my time, I went into autopilot mode, sleeping little, constantly keeping an eye on Karen, forced to relate to her like I would an infant.

In the midst of this hurricane, we drifted into the storm's eye, where the winds were fairly calm, just in time for an important event: Ryan's graduation from the Salt Lake Community College the evening of May 9, with an AA degree in Airframe & Powerplant Mechanics (A&P). With this degree and certification from the FAA, he could pursue jobs working on airplanes and helicopters. He had worked hard to reach this goal, taking classes at the community college during the days, while working the swing shift Monday-Friday at FedEx's Ground sort terminal in Salt Lake City.

Karen and I were very proud of him. It was a huge accomplishment, something to celebrate, and we wanted to honor him by showing up. Fortunately, Karen was unusually calm that day, which allowed us to sit through an extremely long ceremony and take pictures afterward. The "calm winds," another Providential gift, literally only lasted through the night, as Karen's condition declined rapidly in the days that followed.

*****

On the day of the appointment, I lied to Karen, telling her we were going to the Huntsman to see Patrick, otherwise she would never have gone. After I helped her get dressed and into the car, we were off. In calmer days, once there we would small talk with the staff, relax in the waiting area, and then chill out in the exam room until Dr. Jensen appeared.

Not this time. I asked one of the MA's to put us directly into the exam room. Even though we were sitting together, her agitation and frustration started to boil over because I was not able to understand what she was saying or attend to her requests.

One of our favorite medical assistants came in the room to take care of preliminaries. I explained the situation and used her presence to duck out to use the restroom. When I returned, Dr. Jensen had shown up.

He turned to me and said, "I have been with Karen only a couple of minutes and know what the problem is. She is perseverating. The left frontal lobe was traumatized by the radiation, exploding tumor, and resulting blood flow, which caused her cognition and vocabulary to decline. Repeating a handful of words – perseverating – is one of the common symptoms of impairment in this lobe."

He explained that the left frontal lobe controls important cognitive skills such as emotional expression, problem solving, memory, language, judgment, and sexual behavior. Essentially, it is the "control panel" of an individual's personality and communication. The trauma to this lobe, caused by the recent SRS radiation and blood flow, was impacting the central control of Karen's brain. In electrical terms, critical neurological functions were short-circuiting.

While Dr. Jensen is generally quite cautious about getting out the knife and cutting around in the brain, the strategy of "watching and waiting" was not working. The steroids were not working. Karen was a mess; I was absolutely beside myself. Both of us were losing our minds. We were at a crisis point.

Surgery, to relieve the pressure caused by the blood flow, was the only option. To my great disappointment, His week was already filled with other critical cases, which meant the soonest Karen could get into surgery was in one week.

Seven full days!

Oh, no.

My heart sank.

I immediately said, "Yes, we will be there," yet as Karen and I drove home, I knew this would be an impossible assignment, without a doubt the toughest seven days of my life.

I had to watch Karen closely 24/7, as her behaviors were only getting more unpredictable and extreme. For example, she would randomly urinate on the kitchen linoleum, and much worse, on the bedroom carpet. I finally had to get her adult diapers and then force her to use them.

She tried to cook, which I could not allow because of the risk of her burning herself, or walking away, leaving the burners on. One particularly tough day, Karen became very, very agitated when I told her she could not cook. We wound up fighting in the kitchen, pushing and shoving, she trying to get to the range, me pushing her away.

Over many years of marriage, I had never, ever pushed my wife. It was a terrible feeling. Terrible. Eventually, I went outside to the house's electrical panel and turned off the circuit breaker controlling the electric range.

Tasks that Karen would normally do, even with immunotherapy, radiation and surgeries the last six years, were no longer safe bets. For example, one day she told me she was going downstairs to do a load of laundry. At that moment she appeared "normal," and not thinking anything could go wrong, I let her go.

Alone.

Later, I went downstairs to check things out.

To my shock, Karen had jammed our washing machine with clothes, lots and lots of them, to the point where the tank was full of water, but the agitator was not even turning. The only sound was the washer's motor, struggling to do its job, the only smell, the motor's drive belt slipping and burning under the weight.

Because she was oblivious to anything wrong, there was no point in getting mad, or trying to explain why those clothes would not wash. Mostly, I was heartbroken.

Keeping one eye on her, I emptying out half of the washer, dumping armfuls of wet, unwashed clothes temporarily in the basement's bathroom tub, and wound up running 2 ½ loads of wash from the one load Karen had attempted.

From that experience, I made a note to myself: Don't assume anything.

Did I get help?

Yes, sometimes.

When he was home, Neil would flag me when he spotted something wrong and I would take it from there. Amber, although living thirty minutes away and working two jobs, came over whenever possible. Allene lived seven hours away, in Oregon, just across the river from Boise, Idaho. Ryan worked full-time at FedEx and, now done with college, was busy preparing for his FAA exam. My aging in-laws lived in Southern California.

I might have reached out to out-of-town friends for help, but this perseverating/cognitive impairment came on like a thunderstorm, leaving me stunned and behind the power curve. Because Karen had many close calls over the last seven years, it was quite reasonable to think that this complication, albeit stressful, was just another one, so why push the panic button calling in people from distant places?

*****

One day I called Patrick, Karen's friend and Huntsman Wellness Center exercise trainer, asking for his help. Karen had steroids to take and an appointment with Dr. Grossmann in just a few days, but she was no longer cooperating with me. Dr. Grossmann was well aware of Karen's perseverating condition and was quite concerned. Would Patrick help me lure Karen into an exam room?

"Yes, of course. I will do whatever you ask."

My plan was to bring Karen to the Huntsman using the ruse that she would see Patrick for some exercise, when in reality he was going to, 1) firmly instruct her to take her steroids, since she respected him and might listen to his request, and 2) walk her down to Dr. Grossmann's clinic, join us in the exam room, and stay there until the appointment with Dr. Grossmann was over.

Patrick, Dr. Grossmann and his staff, and I carefully worked out the details. On the appointed day, Karen was excited because I had told her Patrick wanted to see her. She could hardly wait. When we got to the Huntsman, Patrick met us, spent some personal time with Karen in the cardio exercise room, and then offhandedly asked her if he could walk down to Dr. Grossmann's office with her.

I fell behind while he walked beside her. Even with Karen's limited cognition, Patrick did his best to emphasize how important it was for her to take the steroids. Although she seemed to listen, I doubted whether anything made sense to her.

When we reached Dr. Grossmann's clinic, staff led us directly into an exam room, bypassing the check-in desk and waiting area. Dr. Grossmann, a nurse practitioner, registered nurse, social worker, and of course Patrick, were all there. Within minutes, Dr. Grossmann knew that surgery was the only option. I agreed to get Karen on the schedule for a PET scan and appointment with him after she recovered from surgery.

Everyone cared deeply for Karen.

And me.

*****

Thursday, May 23, 2013: The day before surgery, I brought Karen to the University Hospital's surgical center for the standard, pre-operation physical exam. Allene and Amber joined me. Their presence was immensely helpful and encouraging.

While the three Swan ladies sat in the lobby together, I slipped back to brief Karen's nurse about her perseverating behavior, where we worked out a plan. The nurse would ask Karen a question, then look over to me to confirm Karen's answer. This would maintain Karen's role as the patient while keeping the process running along with accurate information.

Soon, surgery staff called us back for the exam/discussion. While Karen was struggling to communicate, she was relatively calm. This nurse was a real pro. After the physical exam, she started going through a multi-page checklist. She addressed Karen directly; more often than not, Karen would answer "NO" in a very strong voice. The nurse then looked over at me for the correct information.

Karen never seemed to know what was going on. My daughters, of course, did. The plan had worked. This surgery intake area was where we would bring Karen the next morning at 8 a.m., initiating the surgery preparation process that had become all too familiar.

With that information, we went home, to just a few more hours of managing the agitation and perseverating, after which Karen would be better. At least that was my hope and prayer. Frankly, I never entertained any other outcome. We had been through so much that this looming surgery was just another large boulder in the rushing river that we had to navigate around.

*****

Day of surgery: May 24, the Friday before Memorial Day weekend.

Karen and I got to the University Hospital early. We hung out in the large, recently remodeled lobby, waiting for my daughters to join us.

I had not put an adult diaper on Karen for this transition, thinking that staff would soon have her in a hospital gown and all would be well. That was a mistake. As we waited, Karen urinated as she sat on one of the vinyl chairs, soaking her underwear and skirt, urine pooling on the chair seat. She was not even aware she had done so.

By then, Amber had arrived. Together, we led Karen into an adjoining restroom, where the two of us rinsed the urine residue from her legs and feet, and then I put on an adult diaper I brought in case of emergency…. the one that had just occurred.

After we got back out to the lobby, I flagged down hospital janitorial staff and explained what had happened. They immediately responded. Soon the chair area was blocked off.

That over, Amber, Karen and I walked to the elevator, up to the surgery center. While we waited in the lobby, Amber took Karen to use the restroom again. While in there, Karen lost her balance, Amber could not catch her in time, and she fell, hitting her head.

We all felt terrible about this, especially Amber, but there was nothing she could have done. Karen did not even remember the fall.

The wait was short, the check-in process efficient and calming. Karen, in her bed, plus Amber, Allene, Neil and myself, gathered in a small pre-op room. "Hospital time" had kicked in, so we just hung out in the small room together, talking, dozing, sipping coffee, and hugging Karen. Ryan dropped by for a few minutes before heading off to study.

Eventually Dr. Jensen arrived, and the anesthesiologist after him, explaining what they were going to do. By now, I knew the story they would tell. My children, on the other hand, benefitted from hearing the surgery plan directly from the physicians themselves.

Finally, things kicked into high gear. Karen was on the move, the four of us walking beside her as staff wheeled her bed down the halls. After saying our goodbyes and sharing hugs all around, they whisked her into a surgery suite. It was late morning.

Surgery was scheduled for four hours, so Allene, Amber, Neil and I headed over to the Huntsman's Pointe restaurant for a meal. After that, Neil went to work down the hill on the University campus, while my daughters and I hung out in the surgery waiting room. It was a comfortable enough place, filled with family and friends anxiously awaiting news on their loved one's status, just like us.

Killing time.

Lost in thought.

Mindlessly staring at the TV.

As Allene, Amber and I sat there, I texted family and friends all over the country.

Please pray!!!

Karen is in surgery!!!

When the heart is heavy, four hours seems like forever. Finally, surgery center staff called me to the desk, telling me that Karen was out of surgery and Dr. Jensen would be out to talk with us.

As promised, he was, telling us that the surgery was successful. He had good access to the tumor area, draining fluid and removing residual tumor tissue. The sources of pressure were out of Karen's brain.

Now, she was in recovery.

We could see her very soon.

The important news was that she was alive, responsive, and coming out of anesthesia. Everything else was icing on the cake.

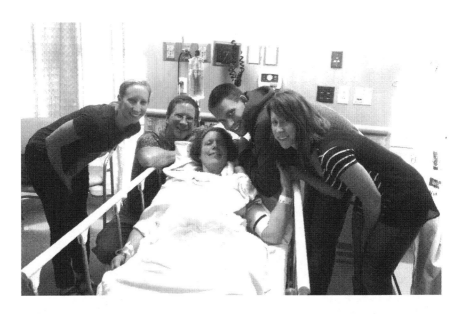

University of Utah Hospital 2013 Pre-Op room

~23~

"You Look Like a Million Dollars!"

There she was, Karen, The Exceptional Responder, laying in the surgery recovery area, flashing her signature smile, signaling to Amber, Allene, and I that, yes, she was alive and on the rebound. It was a joyful moment seeing her again.

Skilled hands had done outstanding work on her brain; prayers were heard and answered. Karen's perseverating had ceased. While very fatigued, she was aware of her surroundings, conversant, and thrilled with the presence of family and friends. What a dramatic change from the previous day!

While others in the community remembered those who had died defending their country or celebrated the beginning of summer, the Swan family members spent the Memorial Day weekend camping out in Karen's recovery room. By now, we knew the routine: hang out, eat, read, talk a bit, laugh, and surround Karen with lots of attention, that is, while she was awake, so she could recover quickly and know she was loved.

Like the previous surgeries, I slept in her room each night, our "private suite" invaded on a regular basis by a steady stream of nurses and phlebotomists popping in at all hours, checking vital signs and drawing blood. It was standard post-operation stuff.

Because Karen had fallen in the bathroom before surgery, and stress to the left frontal lobe can affect balance, staff felt she was a fall risk. This meant that even though I, or a family member, planned on staying with her all the time, they had a specially trained person in the room 24 hours a day to help steady her when she got out of bed to use the restroom, take a shower, or walk in the hallway. A team of three people worked eight-hour shifts, literally sitting by her bedside. They never dozed or slept, even on the midnight shift.

After just 24 hours, it was clear to me that Karen was no longer a fall risk. Staff residents working the long weekend were more cautious and wanted to keep an aide in the room for another day.

Although I chose not to fight this battle, things resolved themselves in a rather humorous way Saturday afternoon.

Karen announced that she needed to pee. The health aide asked her to wait a minute while they unplugged the pump that was dripping saline into her IV.

That was not going to happen! Bounding out of her bed, Karen was on her way to the bathroom entrance before the aide knew what was going on.

I grabbed Karen's arm just as the plastic IV tube stretched to its limit, stopping her. Another foot and the needle probably would have come out.

When it came to watching my wife, the stunned aide was out of her league. What kind of patient has brain surgery one day, and then the next bounds out of bed like a sprinter?

I laughed.

This was classic Karen: strong, determined, and quick.

Once Karen settled back in bed, I walked out to the Charge Nurse's desk, explained what had just happened, and asked that they send the aide home. Within a half hour, the aide was gone.

Mission accomplished.

*****

Due to the long holiday weekend, residents ran the swing and midnight shifts even more than normal. Their roles included great responsibility and a steep learning curve. One would occasionally check in on Karen and interact with me. She was recovering well; no caution flags. While I respected them, I was not intimidated. If there was a judgment call, and I thought I knew more than they did about how Karen responded to treatments or recovered from surgery, I would advocate for a different course.

Dr. Jensen dropped in on Sunday afternoon. After one look at Karen, He remarked, "You look like a million dollars!" Those six words rank at the very top of my list of "priceless" physician comments.

I agreed. She did look like a million bucks.

Actually, far more. She was beautiful and amazing.

She continued to break the stereotype of a recovering brain surgery patient. After just 48 hours, her cognitive responses, walking ability, humor, and even appetite, blew everyone away.

All this is why I started lobbying the nursing staff to page the resident, so I could get Karen discharged and home. If there are no residual issues, home is the best place to heal. The Chief Resident on duty Sunday afternoon was playing it cautious and would not sign off on her release. I decided not to push it. We would stay another night, but if things looked good on Monday morning, we were out of there.

There was a potential wrinkle in my plan: Some medical staff suggested Karen would need rehabilitation for neurologic damage caused by the bleeding tumor, damage which might have affected her gait, speech, or other bodily functions. How to resolve this difference of opinion?

An experienced physician from the University's large rehabilitation department agreed to come by Karen's hospital room Sunday afternoon to assess her cognition and muscular functions. He ran her through a number of neurological and mobility tests, activities she thought were nonsense.

Poor guy!

I imagined him thinking: Who was this woman?

Once he completed the evaluation, we walked together out of the room. I advocated for Karen as we stood in the hallway, adding information from her past history of surgery recoveries that I believed supplemented what he had observed. Physicians do not want impaired patients going home too early, but in Karen's case, he agreed that she was making exceptional progress, and rehab – in or out patient – was unnecessary.

Rehab would have involved a lengthy in-patient stay, plus regular outpatient therapy sessions, draining us of scarce time and energy. His decision spared us those complications. It was a gift.

*****

Monday morning could not come quickly enough. Although it was a holiday, physicians were doing their rounds, which fit into my plan. I engaged the attending physician and told him I wanted to take Karen home.

Her vitals are good. She is walking, talking and eating fine. "Please," I said, "sign the discharge authorization. We want her to recover at home."

So he did. After waiting for "hospital time" to work its ways, including paperwork, prescriptions, and follow-up visit instructions, a nurse popped in the room with "going home" instructions. The Finish Line was in sight.

After getting Karen dressed, one of my daughters grabbed a wheelchair, we got her settled in, piled a bunch of her belongings on her lap, and, along with an aide doing the wheeling, headed to the lobby.

In a matter of minutes, we were on our way home.

Again.

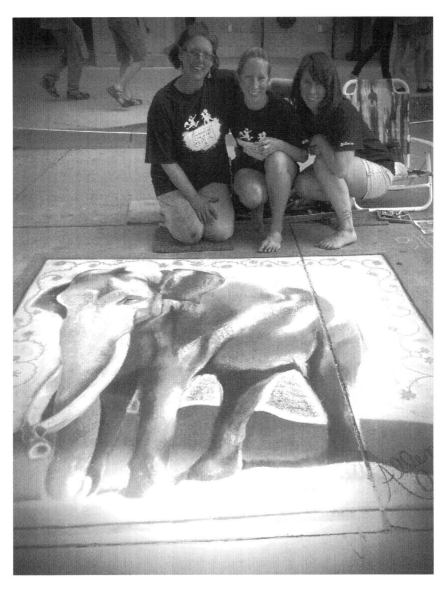

Karen, Amber, Allene – Utah Foster Care Chalk Art Festival 2013

~24~

New Drugs

Dr. Grossmann ordered a PET scan in early June 2013 to assess how things were looking in Karen's chest area, especially the right lung, as the brain surgery's success did not mean that melanoma had taken a vacation. A few days after the scan, we met with Dr. Grossmann. Like Dr. Jensen, he brought the scan results up on the exam room computer monitor for us to see and discuss.

As we feared, there were some hot spots in Karen's right lung, and additionally, several new, small orbs near her the top of her left breast. We discussed how to treat, whether to treat, or watch and wait.

Apparently, the clinical trial drug that Karen had explored down in Southern California two years ago – which theoretically turned a particular cell Off – had recently been approved for general use by the FDA. Karen was not thrilled about using this drug because of the potential side effects, including severe skins rashes and burns for people who did not fully cover up, and the need to use heavy layers of sunscreen while outside. She loved the outdoors; the thought of walking around completely clothed, even in summer, was a dreadful prospect. She might as well wear a tent.

Karen's preferences aside, there was a problem. In Dr. Grossmann's view, we were running out of bullets to stop melanoma's growth in Karen's body. She had used conventional and SRS radiation, surgery, a powerful drug cocktail that included Interleukin via in-patient infusion, and Ipilimumab in the outpatient setting, twice.

All this had slowed down, or suspended, the growth of melanoma for a time, but now it was on the march again. Would this new BRAF-inhibitor drug cross the blood/brain barrier and thereby control melanoma's growth in her brain, along with her lungs? The drug's literature and clinical trials suggested it might.

Dr. Jensen had heard such crossover claims before and was dubious.

What to do?

We wanted a second opinion, specifically Dr. Samlowski's, so in a matter of weeks, Karen and I found ourselves in his Las Vegas clinic waiting area, his last patient of the day. He had already received copies of Karen's surgery report and recent PET scan from the Huntsman, as well as talked with Dr. Grossmann by phone.

We had known Dr. Samlowski for nearly seven years, so we went right to candid discussions when we saw him. His and Dr. Grossmann's opinions on the options were the same, except that Dr. Samlowski suggested that Karen try at least one more round of a drug cocktail which would include Ipilimumab. That was the drug that had caused her so many problems in 2007.

"Absolutely not," was her response.

Did Karen have a death wish? Hardly. The fact was, even for someone as strong as Karen, four rounds of in-patient drug treatment six years ago had been enough. She wasn't interested in going there again.

Since Karen's right lung area had already been radiated by conventional radiation once before, and the tumors were too diffuse to use SRS radiation, there was only one treatment bullet left, the BRAF-gene inhibitor drug. Actually, we learned there were two BRAF-inhibitor drugs, one just released, the other, in the last phase of clinical trials, created by competing pharmaceutical companies. While no drug works for every person in the same way, or at all, clinical trials had shown that these two drugs shrank tumors in about half the people whose metastatic melanoma had a BRAF gene change. In other words, the drug seemed to turn the gene "Off" in a significant number of patients.

No drug comes side effect free. So it was with these two. Common clinical trial side effects included headaches, joint pain, fatigue, hair loss, rash, itching, sensitivity to the sun, and nausea. Less common, but equally serious, were heart rhythm problems, liver problems, kidney failure, severe allergic reactions, and severe skin or eye problems. Some people treated with these drugs developed new skin cancers called squamous cell carcinomas, which showed up on the skin's surface and can often be treated by removing them in an outpatient setting.

Whew, those were some significant side effects. These drugs were not benign, that's for sure. Users beware!

Now that she had the information, which path would Karen choose? We knew that advanced-stage cancer treatment was a series of trade-offs, balancing keeping cancer at bay with managing treatment trauma, side effects, financial costs, and psychological complications. Equally important were one's reasons for being, intangibles such as enjoying life, including family and friends.

Although her concerns about side effects were understandable, especially severe rashes due to even as little as 15 minutes of exposure to the sun, her options were severely limited. Part of the reason Karen thrived for so long was because she loved the outdoors and drew energy from gardening, traveling, skiing, bicycling, hiking, and other activities. Now, with melanoma on the rebound, she was highly motivated to use effective skin-covering strategies throughout the day. That meant full-length clothing, hat, sunglasses, full SPF tint on our car windows, and limiting outdoor activities during the sun's peak radiation hours, 10 a.m. - 4 p.m.

Together, we could make it work.

"I want to try Zelboraf (brand name for Vemurafenib)," she said. "Let's go for it."

Dr. Samlowski started the ball rolling. It was a heavy ball. Coordinating with Dr. Grossmann – keeping him in the loop – was the easy part. The hard part was finding a way to pay for this new medicine. Unlike Ipilimumab, which Karen received in-patient and Blue Cross covered under my medical plan, Zelboraf was an oral medication, which went through my insurance company's pharmacy program. Zelboraf was so new that it was not even on their formulary (approved drug) list, so they would not pay for it.

Pharmaceutical companies anticipate these insurance delays. Because it is to their advantage to get new drugs to patients as soon as possible, Dr. Samlowski sent me to one of his staff, whose sole job it was to coordinate special programs offered by the companies. These options gave patients access to new drugs at either vastly reduced prices, or free, often months before they appeared on formulary lists.

Once back in Salt Lake City, my first task was to fill out the multi-page Zelboraf subsidy application, fax it, and my most recent tax return, back to Dr. Samlowski's staff person, who then faxed it and the supporting medical documentation to the pharmaceutical company. My task was complete; the wheels started turning.

Now we waited.

*****

Since melanoma was not waiting, Karen had a follow-up MRI and appointments with Dr. Jensen and Dr. Grossmann at the Huntsman in late June. When the day arrived, we found ourselves in a familiar setting, an exam room, waiting for the physician.

Although we had been here many, many times before, it never got any easier, especially after melanoma's resurgence. Dr. Jensen, and Melody, his nurse, consummate professionals and wonderful human beings, greeted us warmly and then we jumped right to the meat of the matter, the scan results.

The good news was that the left frontal lobe, the source of Karen's recent perseverating difficulties, was essentially clear. We were grateful. Dr. Jensen's surgical skill was in full view on the computer screen, albeit in shades of black and white.

The bad news was that in the intervening months, three more orb-like tumors had popped up in other areas of her brain, some the size of pin heads, others, pencil erasers (5mm). As I looked at those insidious monsters, it's almost like they were looking back at me, laughing, taunting. Very smart physicians could radiate, cut, and medicate Karen's brain, and people prayed for healing, but melanoma was not giving up easily.

So now there were tumors in her lungs that showed new signs of life, and others in her brain that doubled in size every month. The battle was intensifying. Could Zelboraf restrain or kill the tumors in Karen's brain <u>and</u> lungs? Were its chemical molecules small enough to cross the blood/brain barrier? We would soon find out.

Just a few days after Karen's appointments with Drs. Jensen and Grossmann, I got a call from Dr. Samlowski's insurance coordinator, notifying me that the pharmaceutical company had approved my drug subsidy application. A 90-day prescription of Zelboraf was on its way to our Sandy home via FedEx. At $11,000/month retail, it was "show time" for this new drug.

On a warm July afternoon, the doorbell rang. A FedEx guy stood at my door, wanting my signature. Karen's meds had arrived. Now the ball was in her court, time to take the plunge and swallow the first pill.

The dose was one pill in the morning, one at night. Fortunately, she found the side effects manageable. Even though it was bright, warm, summertime weather, she worked hard covering all her skin with either clothing or a high-quality, high SPF-rated sunscreen and avoided outdoor activities during the sun's peak radiation hours. The occasional headache side effects we controlled with pain medications.

In the early mornings and late afternoons, Karen came out of her house cocoon and lived life, like hiking, socializing with children and friends, gardening, reading, texting folks far and wide, hanging out at the Huntsman's Wellness Center, and going to California several times to see family and her beloved ocean.

Without a doubt, her favorite joy became horseback riding, made convenient, free, and frequent through the incredible generosity of Mim, a fellow schoolteacher and Christian who boarded two horses only five minutes from our home. In many ways, Karen had always been a "horse whisperer," gifted with a sixth sense relating to those large, intelligent mammals. Whether it was brushing their coats, cleaning their stalls, practicing techniques in the corral, or riding in the Wilderness Area, those horses were pure joy for Karen.

In good cancer times and bad, the horse corral and riding became an ideal escape for her and my daughters, whether Mim was there or not. Often, out of the blue, Mim would call or text Karen: Want to go horseback riding today? How about in 30 minutes? Weather was never a barrier; if the opportunity came, they were there.

Off Karen would go, taking the car or riding her bicycle the three miles around the Wilderness Area to Mim's corral. For Karen and my daughters, those horses were hundreds of pounds of comfort and excitement, shared together, outdoors.

What wonderful memories. Thanks, Mim!

*****

The 2013 summer was a transition for several of my adult children. His FAA certification as an Airframe & Powerplant Technician in hand, Ryan decided to move to Alaska for the adventure of a lifetime, driving the distance along the Alcan Highway. He left the day after the 4th of July. We said our goodbyes outside the Draper Great Harvest bakery where Amber worked, and he was off, heading north, way north. Eventually he settled in Wasilla, just outside Anchorage, and quickly found a job with a helicopter company.

Neil was in transition, too. At the end of August, he moved out of his basement room in our home into an apartment owned by the University of Utah. Although a huge step for him, he was ready for it. Karen and I were proud of him.

Whenever possible, Allene drove down from Ontario, Oregon to visit Karen and me, a seven-hour trip if all went well. Amber, although working two jobs, was often over at the house, or if Mim called, mother and daughters would head over to the horse corrals.

*****

An MRI the middle of August showed that Karen's three brain tumors, the ones we were watching, had not measurably changed. A PET scan showed the same stability in her right lung. These results pleased everyone on our medical team.

With that data in hand, it made sense to continue treatment with oral Zelboraf, the BRAF-inhibitor. Perhaps it was the breakthrough drug that patients, physicians, and pharmaceutical companies were dreaming of.

One could certainly hope.

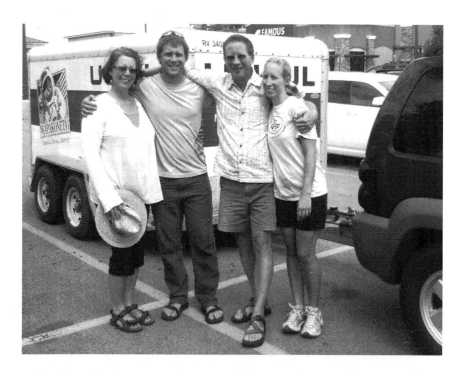

Karen, Ryan, Sterling, Amber – July 2013 – Ryan heading to Alaska

~25~

Transition Months

One day, one memory at a time. We recited this guiding principle often.

Karen was fighting a life-threatening disease and had lived far longer than statistics had forecast. Was there a scientific explanation? Partly. Psychological? Definitely. Something greater? That seems clear.

How else to explain how Karen made it to September 2013, not just surviving, but thriving? While I was extremely grateful for her exceptional care, other forces, supernatural forces, seemed in play as well; acknowledging that was healthy and humbling.

After a long, challenging summer, we were ready for some mental health breaks, and September provided two.

First, Bev and Janet, two of Karen's college friends living in other states, arranged for Karen to join them in Southern California for a week together up along the coast north of the Los Angeles Basin. After meeting up at LAX, they drove to Cambria, a small coastal town north of Santa Barbara, grabbed a large room, and spent four memorable days together talking, laughing, crying, reminiscing, beach combing, eating, and all the other things lifetime friends do together.

Karen loved the ocean. Pictures and texts told the tale, of my wife scampering down narrow cliffs like a mountain goat, heading to small beaches hidden below, and there, digging around in the tide pools. Bev and Janet would eventually catch up with her, telling me later that they were always amazed at Karen's energy, curiosity, and determination. They were supposedly the "healthy" ones, yet she was the first one out of the motel room, and last one inside.

Here she was, living with tumors growing in her brain and lung, yet determined to engage in life no matter what. Maybe she knew something the rest of us did not know or want to admit: Today is the only day she was given?

Bev and Janet told me later that Karen was clearly showing personality-related trauma from all the treatments, but these three friends had known each other since the late 70's, and it didn't matter who had "issues." They loved each other. Period.

Second, after the three friends parted ways, my daughter, Allene, flew down from the Boise, Idaho area and spent a week with her mother near Karen's childhood home in North County San Diego. Photos best told the story of mother and daughter together, mostly spent at Oceanside's local beach/harbor areas, walking along the beach, beachcombing, feasting on the sunsets, drinking coffee, talking, and laughing.

Karen kept herself covered up, using wide-brimmed hats, long sleeve shirts, and lots of pasty sunscreens, since she was taking the Zelboraf, BRAF-inhibitor medicine every day. Even with those limitations, it did not keep her inside, or depressed; she might have had cancer, but cancer did not have her.

This time with Allene would also be Karen's last major outing.

Parting ways towards the end of September, Allene flew back to Boise, while Karen, to Salt Lake City. She arrived home refreshed, full of stories and dozens of wonderful pictures of her dear friends and inspiring ocean. That was a blessed month, and now she was ready, albeit not thrilled, to meet the challenges of more MRI and PET scans coming in early October.

*****

Following scans in early October, Karen and I met with Drs. Jensen (brain surgeon) and Grossmann (oncologist), at separate times, on the same day, which meant that we got to the Huntsman early and left late.

Overall, it was a troubling day.

The good news: data from the PET scan were inconclusive. While there were hot spots in her lungs, the melanoma cell "embers" were just a little larger than the previous scan.

The bad news: MRI images showed new tumors in her brain. Zelboraf was not working, or well enough, in this critical area.

Before the day was up, I was on the phone, arranging an appointment with Dr. Samlowski in Las Vegas. Staff moved other patients around, creating a spot for Karen in mid-October. As we joined him in the exam room two weeks later, he was clearly disappointed that Zelboraf had not stopped the brain tumors. So were we.

There was another option. Tafinlar, a second BRAF-inhibitor melanoma drug, had just come on the market. Although its chemical composition differed somewhat from the inhibitor drug Karen had used over the summer, the strategy was the same: turn off the gene protein that allowed melanoma's rapid growth.

It was worth a try.

Karen, of course, wanted to go for it.

Dr. Samlowski spent an hour with us late that afternoon, brainstorming ideas and discussing which of our limited choices seemed reasonable to pursue. When the three of us walked out of the small exam room, the clinic was dark and empty. We were the only ones left. The three of us exchanged hugs and parted ways.

He would never see Karen again.

We drove north out of Las Vegas, stopping in Cedar City, Utah, along I-15, for the night. The next day, we detoured off the Interstate, heading east and up, into Utah's magnificent red rock country. It was off-season, quiet and cool.

The scenery – sweeping vistas, land uncovered by erosion over millions of years, famous for spectacular dinosaur discoveries – was inspiring and reminded us of the brevity of our lives. This became our last lighthearted road trip together. In many ways, it reminded us of old times, pre-children, when we would hit the road in a 1975 VW Rabbit, exploring on a tight budget.

Fond memories.

*****

Once back in Salt Lake, within days we were in Dr. Grossmann's office, as he had already talked with Dr. Samlowski and was anxious to get Karen on the Tafinlar BRAF-inhibitor drug. While in the exam room, the three of us discussed possible side effects, including reports of severe shaking shortly after taking the drug. Although this was sobering and distressing, Karen had little choice. Her body would soon tell us if this option worked or not.

Fortunately, Tafinlar was in my insurance company's drug formulary, so the Huntsman simply faxed the prescription to the mail-order prescription supplier, and within a couple of days, the drug appeared on my Sandy doorstep. It, too, was an oral medication.

I vividly remember Karen's first Tafinlar dose. She looked carefully at the tablets, looked at me, gave a shrug, swallowed the pills, and took a large drink of water. Then she lay down in bed.

Within fifteen minutes, she was sitting up, hunched over, shaking uncontrollably. I sat next to her in bed, holding her close, trying to comfort her. Her shaking was so intense that I started to shake, too. These two small tablets had created a huge shock effect in her entire body, driving her nervous system to convulse; creating deep shakes that would literally move her, continuously, in lengthy spasms for over 45 minutes.

It was painful.

Distressing.

Exhausting.

Gradually, the shaking diminished and she fell fall back on the pillow, completely wasted, eventually falling asleep from the trauma. Neil, at school, did not have to witness this reaction; it was the last thing he needed to see. While Karen slept, I called Dr. Grossmann's office seeking any possible insight or help. They had no answers, no magic elixir. Some melanoma patients could not take Ipilimumab or Zelboraf without extreme reactions. Karen ran into a similar wall with Tafinlar. We both knew what she had to look forward to the next morning, another dose of the same.

Karen gave it her best shot, but after a week of 45-minute-long convulsions twice daily, she was fed up. One morning she told me, "I am not taking any more."

She was finished.

Done.

Theoretically, she should have tapered off the drug to minimize withdrawal risk. That was not Karen's style; she went off cold turkey. Tapering off drugs was never Karen's style, even in the rare times when I could convince her to do so. She and I picked our battles.

"Dr. Samlowski, Dr. Grossmann," I said in an email later that morning, "Karen is done with the BRAF-inhibitor drugs. What is next?"

*****

I was having problems with high blood pressure, my body's version of a stress response, but I did not want to go to see a counselor/therapist, or just drop in to see an Urgent Care physician. What I really needed was an experienced Internal Medicine doctor who would listen to my whole story and show empathy, carefully diagnosed my symptoms, and suggest possible solutions. In these days of managed care and 15-minute appointments, where was I going to find a doctor to care for me?

In late October, he found me, through junk mail. It was an impossible meeting, were it not for God scripting the details. Normally, I take the junk mail out of my mailbox and toss it directly into the recycle bin. One day, something prompted me to thumb through an eight-page newspaper about activities in my city. In that paper was an ad for Dr. Richard Anderson, an Internal Medicine doctor who was accepting new patients. It caught my eye.

I cut out the ad and set it on my desk. There it stayed for at least a week. Then one day I thought, "Well, whatever, I might as well call."

So I did, explaining to the receptionist that I was a potential new patient and wanted to talk with Dr. Anderson's nurse about his style of practice, experience, age, and whether she would go to see him if she were me.

Fast-forward a couple weeks, where I found myself sitting in an exam room, this time as a patient, in a University Health Care facility close to my home where Dr. Anderson practiced. While new to the area, he had 30+ years of experience running his own solo practice in Burbank, CA, including 20 years as a hospice physician.

After the medical assistant took my vitals, Dr. Anderson walked in, sat down, and we started talking. Ninety minutes later, I walked out of the clinic. Ninety minutes!

I started seeing him every couple of weeks, talking not only about myself, but Karen's issues and how I could "see around the corner" to what might be coming. He regularly gave me 30 to 60 minutes of time, at no extra charge. This went on for months because he was just starting to build up his practice and hence the patient load was light. All the issues I was encountering he addressed in a no-nonsense, humorous way.

Dr. Anderson probably helped me avoid a heart attack…or lose my mind. Six months after Karen died, I came back to see him for a follow-up visit. Although he was glad to see me, he only had 15 minutes to spare as he now had a full patient load. Those large chunks of time he gave me in the fall of 2013 were a unique opportunity never to be repeated.

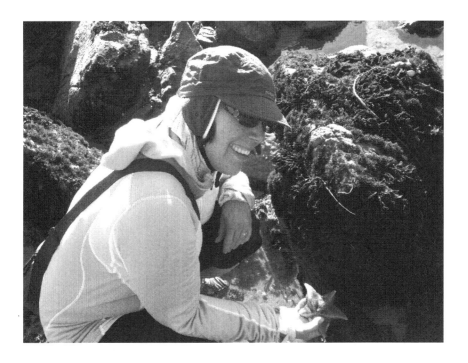

Tide Pools – north of Santa Barbara, CA

~26~

The Seizure

Realistically, the three tumors now growing again in Karen's brain meant that surgery was out of the question. Radiation was the only option left.

Karen preferred stereotactic radiosurgery (SRS); it offered the least trauma to healthy parts of her brain. Drs. Samlowski and Grossmann strongly argued against whole brain radiation because of the danger of cognitive impairment.

Sadly, while Karen's October MRI had shown three tumors of various sizes in growth mode, a mid-November MRI showed not only these three tumors – now doubled in size within the month (some up to 1cm in diameter) – but also three new ones, for a total of six.

What a shock!

The tumors were on a roll, now popping up all over her brain. This was getting out of hand.

Dr. Shrieve, Karen's radiation oncologist, initially opposed using SRS to radiate six tumors at one time, a concern he voiced during the weekly meeting he, Dr. Jensen, and their colleagues held to discuss patients like Karen. He believed that whole brain radiation would have a higher chance of slowing down the growth of the six ones visible on the most recent scan, and new ones not yet visible. As time went on, Dr. Shrieve changed his mind; using stereotactic radiosurgery to go after the six tumors made the most sense.

With that, Karen said, "Let's do it!"

So began the significant administrative process to make sure Karen could get radiation treatment before the Thanksgiving holiday slowed the entire health care system down to a crawl. When the dust settled, Karen was on the radiation schedule for Wednesday morning, November 20, a little over one week before the holidays.

Then life happened.

*****

On Tuesday night, November 19, Karen and I were at the planetarium in downtown Salt Lake City to see an early release of the new IMAX movie, Jerusalem. Prior to the movie, Karen had a seizure as we stood in the theater's lobby, only the second one since her original cancer diagnosis seven years ago.

What exactly happened?

We were carrying on some small talk with a couple of staff members about one of Karen's favorite topics, educating children about science. Without warning, she started slurring her words, causing one of the staff members to look at her quizzically and then politely say, "I didn't understand what you just said."

I looked at Karen's face; she was struggling mightily to get the words out.

They would not come.

In their place came facial contortions, drool from the side of her mouth, and a frustrated, alarmed, and distressed look in her eyes.

I flashed back to September 2007 and instantly knew what was going on.

Karen was having a seizure.

I excused us from the group, grabbed Karen's arm, and walked her over to a corner of the planetarium's large lobby. Sitting with her on the floor, I held her as the seizure spiked, then dissipated about 90 seconds later.

She was exhausted and upset.

The drooling continued, accompanied by an occasional soft mumble. After leaning her against a wall, I ran over to the customer service desk, grabbed some Kleenex and caught the drool in the tissues until the stream finally stopped.

After concerned staff called security, an officer came over to me asking if I needed him to call 911, to which I said, "No, her condition is passing." We sat on the floor together for a few more minutes, and then I helped Karen get up. All totaled, about 15 minutes had passed since the beginning of the seizure.

Once standing, one would have never known anything had just happened. Although Karen had not started talking again, I thought this seizure's symptoms would quickly dissipate, so we headed upstairs to sample finger food desserts provided by the planetarium in celebration of the movie's release.

Appearances are deceiving; something was very wrong. Sitting down at a small table in a corner, Karen looked at me, alarmed and confused. She casually picked up a chocolate cookie, placed it in her mouth, and attempted to chew.

For some reason, her mouth would not work. The bite of food she had taken was stuck between her lips, eventually crumbling and falling out.

Karen looked at me, bewildered. I returned the gaze.

What was going on?

We knew the party was over. I threw away the food, grabbed her arm, and together we walked down to the car parked a couple of levels below. It was time to go home.

Karen tried to talk as I drove us home, but her mouth seemed frozen. Only mumbles came out. Distraught and stunned, it slowly dawned on us that this second seizure, a "simple," one according to medical seizure categories, had affected something in her brain. What did it mean? Could the physicians "fix" this? We would soon find out, the very next day.

As we tumbled into bed, I held her close.

*****

The next morning, Karen could not eat food or drink any fluids. Not only was she unable to talk, we realized that she had lost the ability to chew or swallow. While this was a very serious impairment, we had more immediate concerns on our minds.

We had to get to the Huntsman for the SRS radiation procedure targeting the six evil, growing tumors in her brain. As I drove the 30 minutes, our communication shifted from words to lots of physical touch, eye contact, and impromptu writing. She would write a word or phrase in my ever-present notebook, often with great flourish; I would speak my response, and then she would nod or write more.

Once at the Huntsman, staff led us to an exam room where my son, Neil, joined us. As in a movie we had seen many times before, a young, earnest resident appeared to conduct the standard pre-procedure physical. After brief introductions, I informed her that Karen had a seizure the previous night, and among other things, could not talk. A bit startled, she excused herself, off to consult with her mentors, Drs. Shrieve and Jensen.

When she returned a few minutes later, it was with instructions to immediately double Karen's daily dose of Keppra, her anti-seizure medicine. That was easy. I could do that.

Actually, I couldn't, but would not know it until later on in the day.

Fortunately, even with the seizure, Karen's SRS was still on. Although unable to talk, she was mentally and physically strong enough to proceed with the radiation. It was just who she was.

After so many of these medical procedures, today's routine was oddly familiar, albeit with a new twist. Fifteen minutes before her procedure, I gave her a dose of Valium, this time crushed into fine powder and mixed with applesauce. She managed to force the sauce down her throat by sheer willpower, followed by a swig of water I dropped down her throat as she tilted her head back. Amazingly, she did not gag.

Enough of that white powder must have reached Karen's stomach and entered the blood stream, as by the time radiation staff appeared to bring her to the radiation room, she was in a very mellow mood. We walked together along the winding halls back to the SRS room, holding hands. Neil went back to school.

"It will be about an hour," they said.

I gave the radiation techs Karen's iPod, kissed her, and headed up to the Pointe for some coffee. In just a matter of minutes, the dreaded mask in place, her head fully restrained to the table and body strapped down, and Valium (hopefully) continuing to calm her, Karen would receive targeted radiation to six tumors, the most allowed by the Huntsman in one session.

Once the SRS procedure was over, one of the nurses came out into the Waiting Area and brought me back to an exam room, where I joined Karen for our a post-procedure wrap-up. Like every other time, Karen would get an MRI and see Dr. Jensen in a month. She should take the prescribed steroids until then.

"Call us if there are any problems, " was the nurse's final comment

Standard stuff?

Not!

*****

"Wait a minute," I said to the nurse. "Karen could not talk, chew or swallow. How was I going to get food into her, much less steroids?"

It was Tuesday, the week preceding Thanksgiving, when hospitals, even cancer types, mostly shut down except for the inpatient floors and ERs.

"What was the plan, especially with a big holiday right around the corner?"

"Call this department tomorrow morning if Karen's tongue movement has not returned. We will decide what to do," was the nurse's reply.

Fair enough. With that, Karen and I went home, so she could rest, shake off the Valium effects, and hopefully, regain control of her tongue. We continued with improvised "talking" on the way home. She wrote on a clipboard her comments, fears, and questions in rapid succession, held it up in my line-of-sight, and I then answered verbally or nodded my head.

After previous SRS treatments, once home I would give Karen a strong oral dose of steroids, or at least try to talk her into it. Sometimes she would agree, other times, not. This time around, her impaired tongue made the steroid regimen next to impossible. There was no point in trying. The steroids would just have to wait.

Problem was, Karen had not eaten for 18 hours, and she was already overdue for her morning Keppra anti-seizure medicine. The night was fast approaching when she was due another dose. No food, no steroids, no anti-seizure drug? Things were starting to pile up. We were behind the power curve.

While she could sip water by dribbling it down her throat, chewing was out of the question. What about pureed foods, baby foods? It was worth a shot. I ran over to our local supermarket, headed for the aisle I had not visited in many years, and picked out some pureed proteins, vegetables, and fruit options that I thought Karen might like.

We soon realized that the tongue is an essential muscular organ, not only for communication, but playing a vital role in moving food around in the mouth. How? Initially, the tongue moves food around the mouth so the teeth can efficiently break down the food pieces. Then, the tongue forces that chewed food to the back of the mouth for swallowing. All this is done rather unconsciously while we eat, that is, until the tongue "breaks."

Karen carefully placed small portions of the baby food into her mouth, and using the spoon like an oar, attempted to push the food towards the back of her mouth, where we hoped gravity would help us out. Swallowing a couple small spoons of food, sprinkled with Keppra powder, took many, many minutes. True to her nature, Karen persisted. Once the food was on its way down to her stomach, she followed up with sips of water. On these days, gravity became our best friend.

Wednesday morning rolled around. I crushed Karen's Keppra using two spoons, mixing this white powder into our new "wonder food," the baby food puree. Karen sat in the living room recliner, determined as ever to empty that jar. Like the previous day, it was a laborious, time-consuming process, but it worked. She had triumphed.

Drawing from our experience with Karen's first seizure, I think we were expecting that any moment her tongue control would return. There were huge challenges ahead of us, and a functioning tongue would give us a fighting chance.

That was our reality, all we knew.

We were trying our hardest, clinging to hope.

It was not to be.

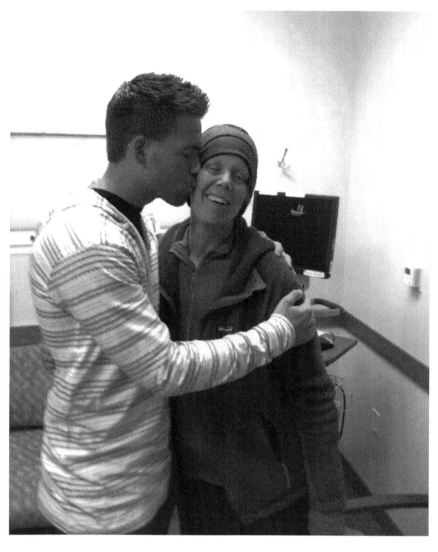

Neil, Karen – Huntsman – waiting for SRS radiation after a seizure

~27~

Thanksgiving 2013

Wednesday afternoon. Two days after Karen's seizure, one after her six-tumor SRS radiation procedure.

Eight days before Thanksgiving.

I called the Huntsman with an update on Karen's condition: she is swallowing baby food, albeit with great difficulty, small sips of water, and ground-up Keppra mixed in applesauce. I have yet to convince her to take the steroids.

Staff on the other end of the phone line offered no magic words or secret solutions, simply because they had none. We were in the midst of a grueling, watching-and-waiting period so common in the cancer journey.

By Thursday, Karen was sleeping fair, eating a bit, doing her best to swallow the Keppra, and getting out with me as much as she could, to run errands and enjoy the fall beauty in our local mountains.

Yes, fall was beautiful, but I was increasingly worried about my wife. So much for controlling my blood pressure! What was driving my concern? Karen was hardly getting 1,000 calories a day, and although we could communicate, with her writing on a tablet and me responding via a clumsy guessing game of talking and/or writing, this was all very stressful and potentially dangerous. The reality was, Karen was suffering from dehydration and slowly starving.

Friday was the same story. Her tongue was still immobilized.

Once we hit the weekend, we were living a nightmare. Karen could no longer force anything but a few spoons of baby food, or even liquid, down her throat, much less a few hundred milligrams of ground-up medications. This was not for lack of trying. My best guess is that less than 10% of what she put in her mouth made it into her stomach. Most of it just dribbled out of her mouth.

By Sunday night, I was desperate. My wife was wasting away before my eyes.

*****

Monday could not have come soon enough.

When the clock struck 8 a.m. I was on the phone calling into the nurses' station in the Huntsman's Outpatient Radiation department, counting on someone, anyone, picking up. I also left a similar message on Dr. Jensen's nurse's direct voicemail line. One way or the other, we had to get help.

Within minutes, Dr. Jensen's office responded. Melody, one of my favorites, was on the line, telling me to bring Karen to the Huntsman Hospital's new Acute Care Clinic (ACC) first thing the next morning, the earliest they could see her.

I dreading another day of waiting, of Karen suffering without food, fluids or medicines, but there was nothing to do but say, "Thanks, we will be there."

Could I have brought her to the ER? Yes, but the ER experience was a consistent downer for us; it was not the place to handle Karen's complex needs.

By Tuesday morning, my dear Karen was very weak. She had gone over seven days without significant calorie intake or fluids, or any assurance that the meds I was mixing in applesauce were getting into her blood stream. In a bygone era, minus what the compassionate staff at the Huntsman was going to do for her on this day, an experienced oncology nurse told me later that Karen would have likely died in a matter of weeks.

On this day, she was not going to die. I bundled her into the car and off we went to our "second home," where we parked, took an elevator up to the Huntsman's second floor, and began walking towards the Acute Care Clinic. On the way we ran into Dr. Grossmann, Karen's melanoma oncologist. I briefly explained that Karen had a seizure the previous week, we were on our way to the ACC, and she had gone 7 days without food.

"I am so sorry, Karen," was his heartfelt response, deep concern written all over his face as he gave Karen a warm hug.

With that, he was gone, on the run to his Clinic to care for other patients. Looking back, I suspect he knew that no matter what the ACC staff was able to do this day, Karen's seizure was likely the beginning of the end.

Because Karen was the ACC's first patient of the day, our wait out in the lobby was short. Once in an exam room, a compassionate medical assistant quickly assessed her needs. Among other things, I explained that she had not eaten or taken in significant liquids for over a week.

Within minutes, Karen was brought back to a larger room and placed in standard hospital bed, where a nurse attempted to insert an IV needle into one of her veins. After several painful, failed attempts, largely due to Karen's dehydration, staff paged a special IV placement team to insert the line.

Providentially, this two-person team was in the Huntsman building, their previous IV line placement had concluded early, and so, within minutes, they were at Karen's bedside. Clinic staff later told me that it was not uncommon for patients to wait several hours for this team's specialized services. On this day, Karen only waited a few minutes.

I stood in a corner of the treatment room watching these professionals go to work on my wife. Using a portable, miniature ultrasound machine, they quickly identified a vein in Karen's right elbow area. Using that image, and experienced hands, one of the team members slowly, carefully inserted an IV needle.

Bulls-eye!

Within minutes, a saline solution was pouring into her body. Staff added a second bag, this one containing comprehensive nutrition in liquid form. Quickly, Karen began perking up. Finally, into the drip line went Karen's anti-seizure medicine, plus an anti-anxiety drug to relax her since the whole morning had been very stressful.

I had a shot of whiskey.

In the midst of all this drama, the ACC physician on duty that day walked into the room. She had already looked at Karen's history online and discussed Karen's condition with Drs. Grossmann and Jensen. Everyone agreed that Karen should receive an evaluation from one the Huntsman's speech therapists. Like the IV team, one was paged, and within minutes walked into Karen's room.

This therapist felt around the outside of Karen's lower head, jaw, and neck, watched her attempts at vocalizing, and observed as she attempted to chew and swallow. Her opinion confirmed our experience; the nerve in Karen's brain controlling her tongue had been somehow pinched, paralyzing that vital piece of anatomy.

Yet, all was not lost. Mixing up a smoothie-type liquid right in front of us, using a combination of apple juice and protein powder, the therapist watched as Karen made a valiant effort to swallow it, one sip at a time. It was not an easy task, even with the techniques the therapist gave Karen, including proper head position, key muscle movements to move the cheeks, and sensations she would feel as the liquid slowly worked its way down the throat.

Karen, determined as ever, swallowed a large portion of the puree.

The room broke into cheers and clapping.

During this cancer journey, when things were at the boiling point, small successes became big deals.

With that small victory, the speech therapist, her colleague, a nutritionist, and the physician all recommended that Karen give pureed foods a try at home, using the techniques she had just learned. It was the least invasive solution. Other options included insertion of a feeding tube through, 1) a nostril, snaking down into her small intestines, or, 2) surgery to insert a port near her belly button, going directly into the stomach.

Karen wanted to try the puree route for a few days. After the saline and protein drip bags finished emptying into her body, and the nurse discussed the doctor's orders with us, Karen and I headed home. She was physically strong once again, her body hydrated and recharged with food and medicine. It had been an exhausting morning, but we were guardedly optimistic.

Once home, I became a blending barista. Into the blender went every type of healthy food I could think of, along with her meds, and then I hit the Puree button. Using the techniques taught to her, Karen was able to get some of the "brews" down, but not without leaning way back in the recliner chair and slowly letting the food drain down into her stomach.

Unfortunately, in spite of our high hopes and Karen's best efforts, the puree approach was not working. She could only get a small fraction of the food I blended past her mouth. Eventually it dribbled back out, caught in the large towel bib I laid on her neck and chest during these feeding times.

Disappointed, it was time to try one of the other options we had discussed at the Acute Care Clinic that Tuesday morning.

*****

Wednesday morning, Thanksgiving Eve

I was on the phone to the Acute Care Clinic at 8:01 a.m., telling staff that Plan A, the puree option, was not working. With Thanksgiving the next day, I insisted that I had to bring Karen into the Clinic with no delay, so we could implement Plan B. Apparently, I had established credibility and trust with the Clinic staff the previous day, because they moved mountains to carve out a time slot for Karen.

"Can you be here in one hour?"

"Yes."

Kicking it into high gear, Karen and I raced around the house getting ready for our now-familiar dash to the Huntsman. Once there, we headed directly up to the ACC, where the medical assistant who had helped us the previous day met us again. Soon, a Clinic physician was in our exam room.

He gave us the raw facts. Running a feeding tube up Karen's nostril and then snaking it down into her small intestines, though less invasive and risky than a port in her belly, was still a significant decision. Not only does one's quality-of-life change, but the body's digestive routine changes, too. In reality, a feeding tube through the nostril is only a temporary solution, especially when melanoma tumors are on a tear in a patient's brain.

The alternative to these two options, to do nothing, was a death sentence. Without adequate food or hydration, Karen would get weaker and weaker and then die. She was not ready to die yet, especially with the Christmas holiday on the horizon, and the outside possibility that the pressure on the nerve controlling her tongue would diminish, allowing her to regain control of her tongue and thus continue the battle with melanoma.

The Clinic physician agreed that a feeding tube, run through Karen's nostril, was the best of bad choices, so I said, "Make it happen."

With that, a series of pieces fell into place, all on Thanksgiving Eve:

- Acute Care Clinic staff expedited the request for insertion of a feeding tube into Karen.

- A physician, specializing in the use of a small x-ray machine needed to feed a very small tube (about the diameter of an earphone cord) down a patient's esophagus to the precise destination, was located, and available, at the University Hospital.

- A Huntsman insurance specialist worked behind the scenes to enlist a preferred-provider company that would commit to delivering all the necessary items for Karen to start her feeding, including pump, formula, tubing and bags, and a trained person who would bring these items to our home that night.

- All of Karen's current prescriptions were called in to the Huntsman's pharmacy, where they translating her tablet medicines (anti-seizure, pain, steroid and anti-anxiety) into liquid form so that I could give them to her via the feeding tube.

- While waiting for the feeding tube insertion, I called Blue Cross to verify that the company providing the formula and equipment was a preferred provider, since we would need lots of nutrient formula, cases and cases of it.

There were many balls in the air that day, lots of people working hard to serve my wife. The critical one, successfully running the feeding tube into Karen's small intestines, was done by mid-afternoon. Following that, we met one last time with the Clinic physician. I told him we were not leaving the hospital until I knew for certain that all the formula and equipment would be delivered to our home that evening.

To put my mind at ease, I spoke directly with the Huntsman staff person working behind the scenes to make sure this happened. She confirmed it, giving me the company's phone number so I could follow up with them directly later in the evening.

With that, Karen and I headed home.

As the sun set, we found the roads packed with folks heading to see loved ones for the long Thanksgiving weekend. Ours would be a long weekend, too, but for entirely different reasons.

So it was.

*****

As I drove, I called the home heath care company that handled enteral care, which is feeding and drug administration via the GI tract.

"Yes," they assured me. "A delivery would be made this evening, and detailed instruction would be provided on dosing the formula, water, and Karen's meds."

"Yes, we are definitely preferred providers with Blue Cross," was the other answer I wanted.

By then, the sun had set. Karen and I were lost in our thoughts, in our car's cocoon, completely exhausted from this day's events, from the last nine day's events. I looked at her, a small tube exiting about a foot from her right nostril, capped at the end to prevent infection.

She looked beautiful.

We pulled into our home's driveway, this time with a more hopeful plan. Plopping down in the living room, both of us dozed. Karen insisted I grab something to eat, so I did.

7 p.m. – There was a loud knock at the door.

There stood a middle-aged man, surrounded by a half-dozen boxes of various sizes. He came bearing "gifts" of nutrient, plus all the paraphernalia necessary to restore Karen's physical strength. My Thanksgiving had come early.

This enteral company employee and I opened up the various boxes, piling the infusion pump, tubes and syringes, aluminum stand and everything else on the kitchen table. Equally important, there was the life-sustaining nutrient, 24 small cans in a case, six cases. Finally, I had the means to regularly feed my wife.

Before Karen and I had left the Huntsman earlier that afternoon, one of their nutritionists met with me to map out how much nutrient, blended with tap water, Karen needed per day. We then translated that data into a number that I would program into the pump's small computer.

That pump "number" in hand, the enteral delivery guy walked me through the entire set-up process: filling the two bags with water and nutrient; getting the pump and line primed and ready to roll; and connecting the line to Karen's feeding tube and pressing Start.

It was a humbling assignment. I was now responsible for the proper feeding and medicating of my wife of thirty-three years, 24-hours a day via the feeding tube. The weight of the responsibility hit me hard; Karen's wellbeing was literally in my hands. Yet, she never expressed the slightest concern about my ability to manage all these details. Her trust in me amazes me to this day.

Apart from an occasional one or two-hour break, once we started down this feeding tube road, there was no stopping, even at night when Karen was sleeping. I divided her daily caloric needs into twenty-four segments and programmed the pump's computer accordingly.

At one point during the pump set-up, Karen turned and gave me The Look, which meant, "Oh, well, here we go again."

More stream rapids and boulders ahead.

More unknowns.

Let's go for it!

There was no one else in the house that night, yet we were not alone. We were never alone.

*****

With that quick, non-verbal dialog over, it was time to take the dive.

I pushed the pump's Start button. Within seconds, the pump drew a 50/50 mix of nutrient and water from the two bags hanging five feet up on the aluminum pole, into a plastic tube about the diameter of a drinking straw. That mix then found its way through a small plastic connector near Karen's neck, allowing the pump line to easily attach to the feeding tube inserted at the Huntsman earlier in the day. From there, the fluids descended into her small intestines.

Did Karen have the sensation that she was "eating?" No, but nutrient and water were flowing into her stomach, fluids that would soon be absorbed and sent throughout her body.

Finally, we caught a break. Karen started eating again.

Prior to her seizure, Karen handled the complex rhythm of the daily medications mostly on her own. I was just a parrot, reminding her if she forgot. Now, since I was her druggist, I needed a system so I wouldn't forget or mess up.

Each liquid medication differed in purpose, texture, and volume. Some required refrigeration, others, not. The feeding tube's small interior diameter meant that I had to learn how to give the meds slowly.

I transformed our main kitchen counter into my medication assembly line, lining the drugs, syringes, measuring cups and schedules up in an easy-to-see-and-follow sequence. No one else, including Karen, was going to do this, so I created a system that worked for me.

"Welcome to the Swan home. Watch Dr. S. Swan as he works his drug and nutrient mixing magic!"

All the dosing was in milliliters. Syringes, into which I placed the various liquefied meds, were as small as 1ml, and as large as 50ml (for the water flush, before and after inserting the various meds into Karen's feeding tube). After using the measuring cups and syringes, I washed them thoroughly and let them air dry in the dishwasher for re-use the next time. Every 4, 6, or 8 hours, I was pushing at least one of those medications into Karen's feeding tube, a routine that occurred around the clock.

Karen and I slept in the same room and bed so I could immediately help her with any problems or toilet needs. When it came to her using the toilet, all privacy was out. This common human routine required that I get up from bed, unplug the pump from the wall outlet (which kicked in the battery back-up), and walk beside her while simultaneously rolling the aluminum stand into the bathroom. It was an odd sort of slow-motion dance…done when we were only half awake. After she used the toilet, we washed hands together, and then reversed the process back to bed.

Although an impressive, high-tech machine, the pump constantly made a thump-thump noise as it drew the liquids out of the two bags and pushed them through the small plastic tubing into Karen's body. Nonetheless, we both slept that first night, somewhat fitfully, but at least there was a sense of relief that Karen was getting food and meds once again.

The next day, Thanksgiving, was a time to wind down from the previous intense ten days, give thanks for the many known and unexpected gifts we had received, and spend time with Amber and Neil, who were in the area. Ryan was up in Alaska and could not make it home, while Allene, living in Oregon, had already burned a lot of leave time earlier in the fall – regularly coming down to spend time with her mom – and was not able to join us.

A friend had given us a gift card to Whole Foods, so we bought some light finger foods there and picked up more traditional stuff from a local Marie Callender's restaurant. Of course, Karen could not eat the food with us, but that was not the point. We were together, enjoying the day as much as we could. The reality was, there was low-level stress constantly playing as background noise. Nothing could be done about this. That Thanksgiving Day certainly took on an entirely new meaning, of giving thanks in the midst of hardship.

Prior to Karen's seizure and tongue paralysis, it was not unusual for the two of us to head out for a long hike or multi-hour road trip exploring in area. Now, we were adapting to a new routine, largely tethered to the pump. While it was battery powered and somewhat portable, we found it easier to keep Karen's total daily caloric targets in mind, note the medication timing, and then unplug the feeding tube. Unencumbered by the pump, we often went for short walks, errands, and field trips to the Planetarium to catch an IMAX movie, or even up the canyons to saunter on nature trails. An hour "off the pump" was common; sometimes we would stretch it to two.

Karen had cancer, plus these seizure complications, but neither of us was giving up. Life had to be lived.

We gave it our best shot.

~28~

Early December

Because Karen had an SRS radiation treatment a week before Thanksgiving, we were on the Huntsman's schedule in mid-December for a follow-up MRI and appointment with Dr. Jensen. Until then, we waited.

In an odd sort of way, we had settled into a new routine, of life with Karen using a feeding tube. One of our country's secular holidays, Black Friday, came and went without us participating. Our children were either working full time, or in Neil's case, living on campus and attempting to focus on his college studies. More to the point, buying things seemed rather absurd in light of Karen's condition. Doubtless, any one of us would have traded all we owned just to have her return to "normal."

To our great shock and joy, we were only a day into December when a ray of hope appeared. Was this a gift of "normal?" As if someone turned on a light switch, Karen woke up one morning and said she wanted an In-N-Out chocolate shake.

I looked at her incredulously. After two weeks of non-stop nutrition via the feeding tube, suddenly she thought she could swallow a shake?

"Yes, I want a shake," was her patented, confident Karen answer.

What harm was there in trying?

Off to In-N-Out we went.

Still unable to speak, Karen stood next to me as I ordered one chocolate shake.

"No hamburger or fries, sir," asked the employee? "Just a shake?"

"Just a shake. And a spoon, too."

We grabbed a booth, sat across from each other, and I watched in complete amazement as Karen dove into that shake like she had never eaten anything before. In a matter of minutes, the shake cup was empty.

A smile crossed her face, and then she mumbled, "Can I have another?"

Of course! Have a dozen if you want! Happily, I bounded up to the counter and ordered two shakes, one for her, one for me. In fact, shakes all around, for everyone in the restaurant!!!

She emptied the second one before I was even half done.

When we got back to the car to drive home, we just sat there and wept for joy.

Once home, Karen grabbed her notepad, writing that she wanted soup and Jell-O. I had neither in the house, but there was a supermarket only five minutes away. I jumped in the car, raced over to the market, and stocked up with high quality, liquid-only soups and Jell-O packet. I particularly recall the short drive home, as I was in an unusually joyful mood, something I had not felt in quite some time.

While the soup warmed up in the microwave, I made one package of Jell-O, setting it in the refrigerator to harden. I was wondering how Karen might handle something warm, or if a cold shake was her limit.

I brought a small bowl of a hearty yellow squash soup on a tray to Karen, who was sitting, relaxed, in the living room. She picked up the bowl and drank the entire contents.

"Is there more?"

There was more, plenty more where that came from. She took a second helping, and then a third.

What was happening here?

The Jell-O set up in a couple hours. I placed a small amount in a bowl, the bowl on a tray, and brought it out to the living room where Karen was sitting. She grabbed the spoon, and in less than a minute, the Jell-O was gone.

"Is there more?"

Of course! Plenty.

I filled the second bowl completely full.

She ate it all.

Pure joy...from Jell-O! Sounded like a T.V. advertisement.

Was Karen's body playing a joke on us? Might this just be a one-day event? A trend?

We did not know.

I had to act on what I was seeing with my eyes, which was that my wife was swallowing a wide range of soft foods today with little effort. That evening, I borrowed a neighbor's micro-blender and started experimenting with all sorts of hot and cold, smoothie-like brews. For example, potatoes could be cooked and blended? Who knew? So could all sorts of vegetables.

Into this liquid I poured Karen's meds.

Why not?

She ate everything I blended.

One day led to another, with Karen eating more and more of every type of blended food. Feeling like things were on a roll, we decided to head back to the Huntsman so the speech therapist could figure out what was going on. If she was swallowing, could the therapist help her talk? Karen was placed on the schedule the very day I called. Better yet, Amber joined us at the appointment.

Once in the exam room, Amber and I looked on as the therapist did a full muscle evaluation of Karen's larynx. She taught Karen some enhanced swallowing techniques, and closely observed as she swallowed some soft food that I had brought along in a cooler.

Impressed, the therapist suggested Karen consider removing her feeding tube. Karen wrote on her notepad: I want to!

After running the idea by staff in the oncologist's office, the speech therapist first carefully removed the many layers of tape on the right side of Karen's face and neck, which had kept the tube from accidentally pulling out of her intestines. Once the tube was dangling free, she slowly pulled the two-foot-long tube out of Karen's body. In a matter of seconds, it was out.

It was celebration time. Joy and smiles filled the room. I only wish I could have bottled that feeling. It had been a long, long time since I felt that happy, for Karen, for everyone.

As preparation for our departure, the speech therapist and a nutritionist colleague gave us detailed instructions for exercises Karen could do with her neck and tongue muscles, and the many types of foods I could throw into a blender to create liquid meals that would taste appealing. It was a daunting task in some ways; Karen had always been the primary cook in our home. Now, the roles reversed. Not only did I need to cook the items, but blend them to create a soupy liquid.

So it would be. I was determined.

Like a victory lap after winning a marathon, Karen, Amber, and I walked around the Huntsman, greeting friends and staff in various clinics and treatment areas. While Karen still could not talk, with concerted effort she could vocalize a few words, and best of all beam her beautiful smile all around.

Oh, could she ever smile, and on that afternoon, we were all beaming with her. It was one of the best days in many, many months.

In addition to the meals I was already blending, I used some of the recipes provided by the Huntsman staff. If one bombed, I tried another. It was actually fun, a nice change from the pump and liquid nutrient humdrum.

Karen could not get enough of In-N-Out shakes. Too fattening? Her oncologist dismissed that concern with a laugh, saying, "If she wants it, she can have it." Karen and I would drive the fifteen minutes to the closest In-N-Out just for a shake. Or two. When she wanted to rest at home, I would have a friend or family member keep an eye on her, and then I would do a quick shake run.

I was ready to do that for the rest of my life.

It was all good.

Until it wasn't.

*****

On the morning of December 5, Karen hit a wall.

She woke up no longer able to swallow.

Anything.

Overnight, something pinching the nerve controlling her tongue had shifted. The "switch" that had miraculously turned on, went off.

Good-bye pureed foods, shakes, and Jell-O.

Melanoma, the emperor of all maladies, had struck back.

It was a body blow.

What now?

Did I consider this relapse an Act of God? Would we only prolong the inevitable by obtaining another feeding tube?

Perhaps.

Yet the tube had given Karen comfort for several weeks, so why not have it inserted again? Over the past seven years, Karen had often proven statistics wrong, consequently it was reasonable to think that she could beat the odds once again. As in the past, many of us thought another rebound was possible.

Karen wanted another tube. She was not ready to die.

Yet.

I made some phone calls to staff at the Huntsman, tapping relationships developed over the years, explaining Karen needed another feeding tube right away. This time around, I was not going to let a week go by without her having nutrition, water, and medications.

The next morning, December 6, two days before Neil's birthday, Karen was back at the Huntsman, getting a feeding tube placed in her small intestines. Once home, I immediately gave her the meds that she had missed the previous 36 hours, and then hooked her up to the feeding pump so she could start receiving nutrient and water. In a dark sort of way, the pattern was eerily familiar.

*****

A week later, mid-December, we drove to the Huntsman for Karen's post-SRS brain MRI and appointment with Dr. Jensen. As Karen and I sat in the exam room, waiting, I flashed back to the middle years of Karen's long journey, the no-evidence-of-disease period, when Dr. Jensen, his nurse, Karen and I would celebrate good news coming one quarter after another. In those days, everyone in the exam room was smiling.

Those years were a distant memory; circumstances had changed dramatically. We were no longer under any illusions that the six tumors radiated in Karen's brain the previous month were anything other than melanoma on the march. The intense battle now engaged, we need to know how many had died or were bleeding, and how many others had appeared in the weeks since the previous scan?

As we looked at the scan images with Dr. Jensen on the exam room's monitor, the jury was out. November's radiation had apparently killed some of the tumors; we saw dead tissue, necrosis, where the orbs had previously been. Other radiated orbs showed signs of radiation damage and the dreaded bleeding. We agreed to give melanoma more time to show its hand. Karen would get another MRI right after the New Year.

Her ongoing, post-radiation symptoms – sleep disruption, significant spikes of pain, random personality changes – were what we had come to expect from past SRS treatments. Dr. Jensen once again urged Karen to take her prescribed dosing of steroids, as this was the primary tool to control the swelling and possibly reduce some of the symptoms.

She agreed to try, but we both knew what was in store, some tough days around the house just as the Christmas holidays were approaching. Nonetheless, we would do our best...together.

In the midst of these strong cross currents, there were periods of great joy. Two events stand out:

~ Following his fall semester final exams, after a three-year hiatus, Neil told us he wanted to start playing the piano again. We were thrilled. Karen and I gave him a budget, told him to check out options, and let us know. Within days, he had an electric piano picked out. A few hours later, he became the proud owner. He and I brought the boxed-up instrument to his University apartment, where he set it up and sent up pictures.

Once back home, I showed Karen pictures of the piano, still in pieces, laying on Neil's apartment floor awaiting final assembly, at which point she pounded her chest several times with her right hand, her newly adopted way of expressing joy. Later that evening, Neil sent us pictures of the assembled piano in a corner of his bedroom.

When she saw those, she started weeping.

~ During December, Karen and I made several trips to Clark Planetarium in downtown Salt Lake City to see three impressive educational IMAX movies: Jerusalem, Rocky Mountain Express, and Monarch Butterflies. Because we were Planetarium Members, we could see the films as often as we wanted, free.

It became one of our most memorable "Date Night" outings together. We sat in the same theater seats, held hands, and drank in all the spectacular 3-D images. For Karen, those images became metaphors of her cancer journey, and in a very personal way, the step to Heaven that she would soon take. She particularly responded to Jerusalem, often pounding her chest during the 50-minute 3-D film, a physical expression of joy, affirmation, and anticipation. To this day, I can still hear the "thump-thump" sounds and "see" her body language in my mind's eye, as we sat together in the dark, nearly empty theater.

This chest pounding was one of Karen's main ways of expressing her feelings – both joys and sorrows – primarily in private settings as she and I sat in our home's living room (me talking, she nodding agreement/disagreement and/or writing comments on a notepad), in the car as we drove around, or at the IMAX theater.

The blows of sorrow were the pain she felt knowing she would soon leave her children. With a mother's instinct, she knew that her beloved children were, in their own ways, confused, sad and hurting, as they watched their mother decline over many years. She sensed their hurts, and it grieved her deeply.

Pounding her chest was an expression of joy and pain. Those "thumps" haunt me even now.

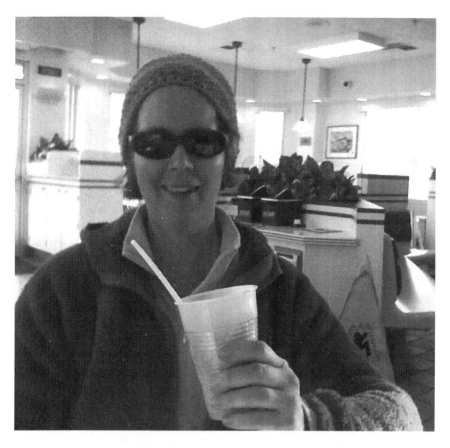

Karen eating a chocolate shake

~29~

Christmas 2013

While the world was racing towards Christmas, with its mix of secular and sacred activities, Karen and I did our best to reach for joy each day, like walks around the neighborhood, drives up the local canyons, visits from family and friends, and even sorting through old pictures.

One unexpected visit a few weeks before Christmas, by Jeff Nellermoe and his wife, Mim, would result in an incredibly close, Providential relationship that continued through the day of Karen's death and beyond. In a truly miraculous way, our lives were merged together that afternoon.

Jeff, senior pastor of a local church, and Mim sat in our small living room talking excitedly about the new direction in their lives. Then, they knelt together beside Karen's recliner chair, praying for her, anointing her head with oil, and embracing her with deep affection. It was another "moment" that is burned in my memory. In the midst of the Swan family's race down a turbulent river, came astounding love from two compassionate human beings just when we needed it.

*****

By mid-December, Neil and Amber descended on the house to set up our artificial Christmas tree; minimalist, compared to earlier years, but at least it was up. There was also a new decoration, a little girl's dress.

A what?

During a recent Costco trip, Karen had spotted a cute little girl's holiday dress – red velour with white-collar – the kind children wear at Christmas church services and other holiday events. She motioned to me that she wanted one. The size fit an eighteen-month-old infant. After a few seconds of internal hesitation, I agreed.

Once home, Karen wrapped a string around the stairs banister in our living room and hung the little red dress from it. Like a giant ornament, the dress symbolized Karen's love for her daughters, reminding her of when they were that small. A couple of days later, Karen wrote on a notepad: I want another dress!

I briefly thought to myself, "Really, another dress?" Thinking done, I left for Costco, part of me hoping they were sold out; part of me hoping there was another identical one on the rack.

There was! I grabbed it, along with a couple other food items, and headed to the front to pay. Several women approached me, commenting on the cute dress and asking why I was buying it. I gave the short answer, that my wife wanted it for her daughter.

*****

Even with Christmas just around the corner, I tried and tried to arrange a way for Karen to see Dr. Samlowski down in Las Vegas. I had been keeping him informed about Karen's brain, lungs, and feeding tube conditions via email. He was quite concerned about her and anxious to explore other treatment options, to the point of moving other patients around in his schedule just so that he could see her. His loyalty and love for Karen were simply unmatched.

Unfortunately, try as I might, I could not figure out a way to make the trip happen. Karen's physical and mental condition was just too brittle even for flying. Mine, frankly, was not much better.

It was a sad moment when I finally emailed Dr. Samlowski that a Vegas trip was impossible, at least before the end of the year. Would a trip before Christmas have made a difference? We will never know.

Three days before Christmas, December 22, Karen's feeding tube caught on something at home and, as she moved, completely pulled out of her body. She came to me holding the tube in her hand, a sheepish expression on her face. We laughed, and then the "Resourceful Me" kicked in. Much like the recent pre-Thanksgiving drama, I knew we needed to get Karen back to the Huntsman promptly so they could run another tube before the place functionally shut down over the long holiday.

As in the past, I tapped the Huntsman relationships Karen and I had built over many years, bypassing the general phone switchboard and calling directly into her oncologist nurse's phone.

That started the ball rolling. Within 24 hours we were at the Huntsman's Acute Care Clinic, going through the preliminary exam and waiting for a slot later that morning to have another tube placed. Fortunately, the procedure went without a hitch, and we walked out of the Huntsman given another chance to celebrate Christ's birth together without the added stress of Karen suffering malnutrition and dehydration.

Like so many times over the past seven years, we reminded ourselves that it was one day at a time. That is all we were given.

Within it, we lived life, challenges and all.

*****

Overall, this would be a low-key Christmas season. Ryan was hard at work in Alaska, as was Allene in Oregon until Christmas Eve. Karen's extended family remained in California, and my sister, a widow, was spending time with her four children. Had we known then what we knew in March 2014, I might have strongly encouraged Ryan to join us, even for a day or two. Yet, we had no way of knowing. This 7+ year cancer journey had faked us out so many times before that we could not guess what was around the corner, much less what would happen in less than three months.

Allene arrived home on Christmas Eve, and together with Amber and Neil, we went to a local church's Christmas Eve services. Any time Karen went out, I had to adjust her nutrient and meds schedule for the hours spent off the pump, rearranging the calculations once we got back home. These occasional outings were important, but we didn't do many because of the logistics and fatigue.

Christmas day came. The Swan's theme: keep it low-key.

We exchanged presents.

My daughters made a simple meal that the four of us ate in the living room so we could all be with Karen.

Ryan joined us for a few minute via Skype.

I dragged everyone outside for some impromptu pictures, capturing priceless images of Karen and her family around the snow-covered ground before we were shaken to the core the next month.

After Christmas, Allene, Amber, and Neil returned to their homes and jobs, leaving Karen and I to our "normal" daily routine of feedings, meds, times together in the living room, and occasional outings. It was during the week between Christmas and New Year's that I realized I had burned out, my "being" exhausted in every way. I had pressed hard from Thanksgiving to Christmas, but after those big events, I let my guard down and the collapse, mainly mental, came.

And I did not know where to turn: not to my children, who were exhausted themselves; not friends, who were knee deep in holiday celebrations, and some unsettled by evil cancer; and not extended family, who had their own time demands, sense of priorities, and widely varied responses to Karen's illness.

Like a light coming on, a name jumped out at me: Rose. She was one of Karen's two sisters, living in Southern California.

I called Rose and her husband, Bill a couple of days after Christmas and appealed for their help. Within a matter of a day, they had bought her a plane ticket, in the midst of one of the most expensive times of the year to travel, so she could come serve and love us when we really, really needed it. Rose arrived on December 30 and stayed a week.

Karen and I drew strength simply from Rose's presence, from "being there." Her tangible gifts of time, care, and laughter during those intense days are what love is all about.

*****

Like Thanksgiving and Christmas before it, New Year's Eve was rather quiet at the Swan home. Although lightly snowing, Karen, Rose, and I decided to drive up Little Cottonwood Canyon, just a few minutes from the home. Because Alta is located at 8,500 feet, we dressed warmly and found a spot to park facing the mountain's north face, right along the side of the narrow, two-lane canyon road. It was a spectacular night: celebrations going on down near one of the lodges; snowflakes drifting down from the darkened sky; colored lights reflecting on the snow covering the ground.

Then came the fireworks, popping above the ski area, briefly illuminating the dark mountains and creating echoes that slowly wandered down the canyon. After that, the torchlight parade started half way up the mountain, involving hundreds of skiers with red flashlights in their hands, snaking their way in a long, serpentine chain down to the base. Finally, there was the ski patrol's impressive decent from a crevice near the peak of one of the mountains, this time with white torches. They came down quickly, with great finesse.

The three of us were absolutely mesmerized. Karen, a bit chilled, remained in the car during the celebration; throughout the various events she pounded her chest with her right hand. It was a spiritual experience for her, she wrote me later, a Heavenly vision, sensing that an even greater drama was close at hand.

Once home, like other nights, our Karen-going-to-bed routine kicked in. No staying up until midnight, ringing in the New Year for us!

Getting Karen ready for bed involved many steps:

First, Rose and I helped her use the toilet and change into flannel pajamas.

Second, we cleaned her teeth by dipping a warm washcloth into mouthwash, rubbing the cloth all over her teeth, and then carefully rubbing the cloth on her tongue and sides of her mouth.

Third, while Karen sat up in bed and Rose kept her company, I went to the kitchen. Using syringes of various sizes, I drew liquids out of the various prescription containers, placed everything on a large plate, and headed into the bedroom to give her the medications that would begin the overnight routine.

One by one, I pushed the meds into her feeding tube, each time flushing the prescriptions down with 10-15 ml of tap water, concluding it all with 25 ml to make sure that every last drop made it into her GI tract.

Finally, in addition to the mandatory meds, if Karen seemed agitated or I thought might fight going to sleep, I would give her a dose of Lorazepam, which is a sedative/anti-anxiety drug. Once that kicked in, she normally was asleep within the hour. While there was no guarantee that she would sleep through the night, at least the two of us started out the night with rest.

Once those meds were in her system, I headed back to the kitchen to prepare her nutrient for the overnight period. First, I poured four cans of Promote nutrient in one bag, and an equal amount of tap water in the other. After priming the infusion pump, I rolled everything into the bedroom. The stand stood right next to Karen's side of the bed, close to an electric outlet, and equally close to her pillow, allowing slack so she would not roll in her sleep, potentially pulling out the tube.

Sitting on the side of the bed next to her, an electric blanket keeping her nice and warm, I wiped the port end of her feeding tube one last time with a disinfectant, plugged the male end of the pump line into her tube, started the pump, and with that, we were done.

Almost.

The very last step of this process was the most memorable for me. I often grabbed a chair and sat next to Karen, holding her hand as I talked with her about the day; of memories of our lives together; of our children and extended family; of what might lie ahead; of Heaven and Jesus. Often I would pray, or sing some of her favorite songs out of a hymnal. Once she started drifting off to sleep, I read quietly until I could hear her lightly snoring.

Alternately, if I was particularly tired myself, rather than sit next to her, I put on some of her favorite music. Together we had created several playlists, instrumental music that included violins and cellos, or Christian vocal music that gave her hope and peace. This music had a profound, calming effect on Karen's spirit, lulling her to sleep in no time. It was better than a drug.

Once she was asleep, I headed back to the kitchen to clean all the syringes, throw a load of hand towels in the laundry – which I used as bibs when I gave Karen her meds during the day – and then headed for the living room to chill out.

On this particular New Year's Eve night, I talked with Rose for a few minutes, and then headed to bed, joining Karen, who was sound asleep. Within seconds, I, too, was in dreamland.

*****

2 a.m. - Time for another medication dose.

If I did things right, Karen would not wake up, even though I stopped the pump, unplugged the line from the port near her neck, pushed in the meds and tap water, and then restarted the pump. After weeks of practice, I could do this routine when I was half asleep. I only needed to fully concentrate as I drew various medications out of the prescription bottles into the syringes.

6 a.m.

Same thing, only this time I added more nutrient into the feeding bag, because the previous night's volume was already in Karen's body. Ideally, Karen would stay asleep.

The wild card in our nightly routine was her bladder. When she needed to urinate, I helped her by unplug the pump, walking beside her, shuffling into the bathroom, and cleaning up after she used the toilet. I don't know how to explain it, but whenever Karen got up from bed to use the toilet, I instantly awoke and met her on her side of the bed, often before she had completely stood up. This "small thing" was a big thing, one of many, many reminders that my caregiving service was not accomplished just by my human power.

So it went, day in, day out.

*****

After a week serving my family and providing loving companionship to Karen, Rose flew back to California. Before she left, I called Gail, another one of our amazing friends, asking her if there was any way she could fly out to help me for a week.

"I will be there," was her response. "When do you need me?"

"As soon as you can get here."

It would be two weeks before Gail arrived. During that time, Karen and I came to the sobering realization that the feeding tube was only a temporary fix. It did not solve the cancer problem, only kept her from starving to death. Something would have to give.

It soon would.

Whether someone was there to help me or not, the nightly pattern of getting Karen "settled" for bed – nutrient, meds, recorded music, Bible reading, singing hymns, etc. – continued.

One day blurred into another. After Karen fell asleep, I often would walk out to the front porch, gaze up into the Heavens ablaze with thousands of suns from distant solar systems, and plead with God.

"Heal her, please!"

"Take me, not her!"

"Why this, why now?"

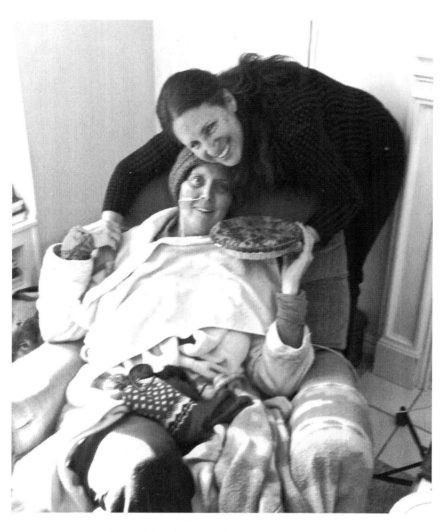

Karen, Rose Zellmer (sister) – Sandy home

~30~

"Candor is What We Want"

After the holidays, Amber and Neil, our children living in the area, often dropped by to spend time with Karen and give me breaks. These two were a sight for sore eyes, no matter how long they stayed.

If Karen was up to it, she and Amber would head over the horse stables, either to rub down the horses, or better yet, go on a trail ride together. Although these types of outings were challenging from a feeding & fatigue perspective, they were essential for everyone's mental health, so the trade-off was absolutely worth it.

Soon Gail arrived, and like Rose before her, was there to serve Karen, my children, and I. Often people ask what they can do when someone is ill? Rose and Gail lived the answer. Show up! Bear burdens. Be present. Love. Laugh. Hug. Cook meals. Clean the house. Give the caregiver breaks.

Just… be… there.

There are thousands of reasons for not coming, but when the family or friend's need is acute, what really matters?

As a treat, Karen and I took Gail to the Planetarium to see the IMAX movie, Jerusalem. Once again, we sat in Karen's favorite section, way up on the top row. I can still see Karen in my mind's eye, slowly, deliberately, walked up the stairs, one foot planted carefully in front of the other, heading to "her" spot, her chair.

She made it.

Gail sat between us, holding Karen's hand the entire time. As the film ended, Karen lightly beat her chest. She knew; Gail and I knew. We were watching a spectacular movie about the city where Jesus walked, taught, and rose from the dead.

It was clear! Soon, Karen would see Jesus face-to-face.

*****

January 13 – Monday
Early light.

I emailed Dr. Grossmann, Karen's Huntsman melanoma oncologist, updating him on where things stood as I saw them, primarily that managing her daily care, personality vacillations, and family stress was finally overwhelming me. I also told him we were going to the Huntsman later that day for an MRI, followed by appointments with Drs. Jensen and Shrieve the next day.

I was desperate.

"What," I asked him, "should I do now?"

His response? He took the ball and ran with it. Without even asking me, he instructed his staff to move other patients' appointments around, carving out a rather lengthy one for Karen the next week, on Tuesday, January 21. I only found out about his initiative on Karen's behalf when his office called me a few days after my email to confirm Karen's visit.

"Karen has an appointment with Dr. Grossmann? I had no idea. Of course, we will be there." When the chips were down and it mattered most, Huntsman physicians and staff were there for us, even when I didn't ask.

Mortality is an unnerving subject, so most of us avoid it. This is true even for cancer patients, caregivers, and family. From experience, physicians know this, so often they hesitate to express the seriousness of a patient's condition to a patient or family members. Although people might look at them as gods, and perhaps some physicians do adopt a god-complex, it's a risk for a physician to suggest that a patient is in their last days.

Perhaps they will rebound?

Maybe they want heroic efforts to cling to life, no matter what?

Sometimes it is as simple as the patient thinking, "If I don't ask end-of-life questions, maybe the illness will go away?"

I recognized many of these common responses to potential death in myself; after all, Karen had lived way beyond the statistical averages, and I had sometimes become complacent, forgetting that melanoma was a relentless foe.

This time was different. Karen's seizure, multiple tumors in her brain, and the gentle but persistent messages from her physicians and nurse practitioners meant one thing: we needed a candid appraisal from Dr. Grossmann.

So now that I knew Karen was on his schedule for the following week, I emailed him back, stating, "Candor is what we want. Give it to us straight. Consult with all your colleagues, including Dr. Samlowski. Look carefully at the scans. We want your frank assessment."

While we waited for that assessment, Gail joined Karen and me at the Huntsman for the MRI. Her presence was invaluable, among other things helping me give Karen liquid Valium 30 minutes before the scan's start time. Before leaving the house that morning, I had placed all the necessary items in a cooler. As the three of us sat in a waiting area, I drew that powerful relaxant out of the bottle with a syringe, slowly squeezed the contents into Karen's feeding tube, and then flushed everything down with tap water.

Ten minutes after the Valium hit Karen's stomach, she could hardly sit up. The drug nearly knocked her out. That was the goal; we could not afford any type of agitation during the scan. There were too many pieces lined up in sequence for that important "picture" to get delayed.

About 20 minutes after I gave Karen the Valium, radiology staff came to the waiting room, indicating it was time for the scan procedure. Even with Gail holding one arm and me the other, Karen was too languid to walk on her own, so we placed her in a wheelchair. Staff then brought her to the scan room, for the last magnetic resonance image she would ever have to endure.

Most people will never have even one MRI in their lifetime. Dr. Jensen told us the next day that in his 25+ years as a neurosurgeon, Karen held the record for the most MRI's of any patient he had ever treated.

The total?

I lost count, certainly dozens and dozens.

Once the MRI was complete, Huntsman staff wheeled Karen down to the first floor. As Gail stayed with her, I retrieved the car. To home we went, back to relax, warm up, and reconnect Karen to her nutrient pump.

*****

January 14, 2014 – Tuesday

Like a yo-yo, Karen, Gail and I piled into my Subaru for the well-worn trip back to the Huntsman.

Once there, we headed to Clinic 2E, at the far end of building, for this very important meeting with two of Karen's key physicians. Along the way, other physicians, nurses, and support staff greeted Karen and I. We had been there so long that dozens of people knew us, cared for us. Strange, but this place had become home.

Amber, living and working close to the Huntsman, joined us in the waiting room. Soon, Barbara, an MA that we had come to know well, called us back to the "vitals" station, where she recorded Karen's weight, temp, blood pressure, pain and general comfort level. As Barb asked the questions, Karen wrote her answers.

Next, it was on to an exam room. "The physicians are on schedule, so it will be just a few minutes," were Barb's parting words.

Within minutes, in walked a fellow, a doctor at the top of the MD-student food chain.

Alone.

I was annoyed.

This exam room was an emotional minefield, and he had just entered blindfolded. We had never seen this doctor before; all that he knew about Karen was from chart notes or discussions with his mentors.

Fellows were often found in complex settings like the Huntsman, mentored by an attending physician while learning advanced diagnostic skills. Today was a very bad day for him to parachute into our lives, especially alone. I was in no mood to let him interact with Karen for very long. Defining boundaries early, I told him Karen could not talk, and this was a critical day because we expected to see MRI results from her primary physicians.

This immediately threw him off; not knowing what to do, he started asking Karen questions. Exasperated, she threw up her arms and loudly mumbled, "I CAN'T TALK."

I intervened, telling him to ask me, since she could <u>not</u> talk, and furthermore, I knew the answers he was asking.

Then he attempted to do a brief physical assessment of her motor skills, neurological response, walking, etc. Karen was getting ticked off, as were Gail and Amber, body language screaming out their collective displeasure. At one point, the fellow asked Karen how well she could walk. She jumped up and literally danced around the exam chair in the middle of the room, all the while shooting the fellow a look that meant, "Don't mess with me, buster."

Stunned, he turned to the computer, intending to show us the results of the most recent MRI scan, at which point I said, "No, you are not going to do that. This meeting and those scan results involve life and death issues. No disrespect intended, but we want to hear the news from Drs. Jensen and Shrieve."

Nodding, the fellow left the room.

*****

A few minutes later, Drs. Shrieve and Jensen came in, along with Melody, Dr. Jensen's nurse, and the fellow, who stood quietly over in a corner of the room, taking notes. I told Dr. Shrieve that we wanted to hear the scan results from his own lips. With that, he had us gather around the computer screen and walked us through yesterday's MRI results.

I had seen enough of these images to know right away that the results were a mixed bag. Some of the radiated tumors were dead, a couple, potential problems (maybe bleeding), and a few new ones had appeared. The exhausting, deadly reality of tumors popping up in her brain was not going away.

We discussed the trends and options.

I asked about the seizure's side effects, most importantly, what could be done about the pinched nerve?

Drs. Jensen and Shrieve looked at each other, unusually quiet; pooling decades of experience, their silence was telling. I looked at Dr. Jensen's body language; I saw resignation. At that moment, I knew the journey was nearing its end game. One idea, admittedly a long shot, bubbled to the surface: use a strong oral steroid treatment for a few days to see if that shrinks the tumor pushing on the tongue's nerve. It was the only option on the table.

I knew how strong steroids would affect Karen's psyche, but what alternative did we have? Karen gave a thumbs-up to the idea, and with that, Drs. Shrieve and Jensen gave Karen warm hugs, shook my hand, and then they left. Karen would never see either again.

Steroid prescription in hand, Karen, Amber, Gail, and I headed down to the basement's parking area. It was a sober time. We were all upset. At one point, Gail said to me, "I am surprised you let that fellow quiz Karen as long as you did. I would have told him to get out of the room right after he asked her the first question." Amber nodded her agreement.

They might have been right. It was my judgment call, in a tense setting. I'm just grateful that Drs. Shrieve and Jensen quickly came into the room after the fellow's departure. We needed to ask the questions of Karen's key physicians, even if the answers meant the end was in sight.

After Gail took several pictures of Karen, Amber, and I as we stood in the parking garage, Amber headed to work, and Karen, Gail, and I drove back home, to familiarity and the ever-waiting nutrient pump.

While driving home, I called my go-to local pharmacy, Walgreens, and asked them for a liquid steroid prescription. By now, both the pharmacists and techs knew me by voice alone and they often moved mountains to help us. Once again, they did. I had the oral medicine waiting for me within the hour.

I started Karen on it immediately.

Karen bravely leaned into the steroid challenge. To help, I gave her frequent doses of the sedative, Lorazepam, which moderated the intense mood swings, but also made her very sleepy. Fortunately, Gail was there to help me help Karen.

Wednesday came: no change to her speech or swallowing.

Thursday: same thing.

By Friday afternoon, the experiment was over; the nerve was still impaired.

Apparently, there were no more bullets to fire at our enemy.

I called Melody at Dr. Jensen's office and told her the steroid option did not work. She instructed us to taper Karen off the steroid and continue with the other meds. Karen had no intention of tapering; she went off the steroids cold turkey. What was the point of proceeding with caution?

Gail spent Friday and Saturday smothering Karen with words of love, lots of touch, and many expressions of spiritual care. She had served us well; it was the last time she would see Karen. She flew home two days later, Sunday morning.

It had been a full week, so Karen and I, largely alone again except for brief visits by Amber and Neil, spent the next two days resting up for Karen's critically important upcoming appointment with Dr. Grossmann.

*****

January 21 – Tuesday, Clinic 2D, The Huntsman

Karen and I, and my insurance company, essentially owned this clinic, since we had been there more times than I could count. The staff all knew us by name, expediting the check-in process. Today, that is where the familiarity ended. Important appointments like this are often scheduled for 45 minutes. Exploring treatment options with the oncologist and his staff just takes time. Although Karen and I were veterans of these appointment sessions, this one would change our lives. We would soon learn why.

Staff brought us to a large, empty exam room, where we sat and waited.

In walked Joan, one of Karen's favorite nurse practitioners. She gave me a long hug, and then walked over to Karen, giving her an even longer one. The two women sat together on the room's couch, ready to support Karen as Dr. Grossmann delivered his recommendation.

I soon realized that her appearance was not random. Dr. Grossman had arranged for several of Karen's beloved staff friends to join us that day, people whom Karen had come to love and trust. Moments later, Kathrine, a social worker, walked in and greeted us warmly. Although new to the Huntsman, she had quickly become a valued source of medical, emotional, and spiritual support for us.

Both women showered Karen with a tremendous amount of love and care. Joan held my wife's hand, as Kathrine stood very close by. Their presence created emotional strength that would help Karen and I cope with what happened next.

*****

There was a knock at the door. In stepped Dr. Grossmann and his nursing team, now making a total of seven in the exam room. For a variety of reasons, Karen and I needed each of these individuals there that day. We trusted them with our lives.

Dr. Grossmann sat down on a short, round swivel stool, placing himself just a few feet away from Karen, staring right at her.

After a few pleasantries, he said, "Karen, I've discussed your situation with all of my Huntsman colleagues, including Dr. Jensen and Dr. Shrieve, and spoke with Dr. Samlowski in Las Vegas by phone just yesterday. In addition, I have carefully reviewed your scans from recent months, and your treatment history these past seven years, including your body's response to the BRAF and immunotherapy meds the last couple years. In light of your brain condition, complicated by the seizure, I recommend suspending further treatments and transitioning into hospice."

With that, Karen began quietly weeping. Joan pulled her close.

For a few seconds, all seven of us were silent. Summoning all the rational strength I could find within myself, I asked Dr. Grossmann to elaborate on his hospice conclusion.

He explained that her brain had been heavily damaged by all the radiation, and further radiation would only make things worse, easily leading to a loss of bodily functions beyond tongue control. In addition, chasing further treatments would be exhausting.

He asked, "Is this chase what she wanted?"

There was a pharmaceutical option, a drug currently in early clinical trials that the Huntsman might get access to…in a couple months. Problem was, based on the trial results so far and even assuming a best-case scenario, Karen's life would likely only be extended by a few weeks.

> Side effects of this clinical trial drug?
> A wild card.

> Quality-of-life by chasing the few weeks of life extension?
> Unknown.

~31~

The Choice

Dr. Grossmann, compassionate and direct, was just what we needed. He summarized the options as he saw them, reiterated his recommendation for hospice, and then asked Karen what she wanted.

"Hospice," she mouthed.

With that one word, melanoma had finally won the battle.

BUT…NOT…THE…WAR!

Karen had won <u>that</u> long ago. She would have to wait a few more months, until Heaven, to hear an accounting of the many impressive, life-shaping victories.

I asked Dr. Grossmann to speculate on Karen's longevity.

His answer? Perhaps two months.

How should we think about the feeding tube? He explained that when a person's body is in decline, liquid nutrient delivered by a feeding tube actually exacerbates issues within the GI tract. Force-feeding a person, thinking that it keeps them alive, actually causes distress.
As he correctly predicted, Karen would encounter this distress in just a few weeks.

He also told us that an experienced hospice nurse would know how to help us manage these feeding issues and inevitable complications. Karen was currently receiving 2,000 ml per day, about 2,000 calories. He recommended we immediately drop that to 1,200 ml/day, and then work with the hospice nurse on a taper plan.

"When should we stop the feeding entirely," I asked?

"Karen will know," he replied.

As our formal meeting drew to a close, I told Dr. Grossmann and the staff that I had a story to tell. I felt it would serve as a fitting conclusion to his care of Karen, the human being he had come to serve and respect. He welcomed it.

Since many in that exam room loved the outdoors, the story I chose was about Karen riding in the SLC Bike Ride in April 2013, scarcely nine months earlier.
- Leaving early in the morning without me
- Driving herself
- Riding in the rain for the sheer joy of it, and
- Arriving at the Huntsman Hometown Heroes Finish Line tent to hear Patrick, her beloved Wellness Center trainer exclaim, "How did you do that?"

"It was," I said, "so typical of Karen."

As I concluded my short story, I watched everyone's eyes shift over to Karen, communicating a profound respect for what she had accomplished that morning, a metaphor, really, for what she had accomplished over thousands of mornings since the fall of 2006. After a few moments of silence, Dr. Grossmann said, "May I have permission to use that story in my interactions with other patients, as I think it will inspire many?"

Karen nodded yes.

Finally, I thanked Dr. Grossmann and his colleagues for their excellent care.

With that, the appointment was over. He stood, hugged Karen and me, and then left the room along with his nursing staff.

*****

Joan slipping out to call Bernadette, another one of Karen's favorite nurse practitioners, someone who had walked beside us from our very first day at the Huntsman years ago. That left Karen, Kathrine, and myself in the room.

That's when I lost it.

I broke down crying.

Hard.

So did Karen.

The last 7 ½ years had been as difficult as anything we had ever faced, but in a strange way, we had adjusted to the treatment roller coaster, the highs and lows, victories and disappointments, close calls and bad news. Now we were veering off that oddly familiar road, to something completely new and foreign, hospice, and minus divine intervention, death soon to follow.

Gradually, stunned silence and exhaustion replaced our tears. It was then that Joan, and her colleague, Bernadette, entered the room. As they did, Kathrine walked me outside to a hallway, so Joan and Bernadette could have some private time with Karen. As I exited, I looked over my shoulder and caught a glimpse of these two amazing women, surrounding Karen as she sat on the couch, holding her, weeping with her, comforting her.

It is an image of caring that is forever seared in my memory. I have little doubt they were angels in disguise, working on assignment at a cancer hospital. They loved my wife. And me.

Standing in the hallway, the Huntsman staff and I discussed hospice options, such as who were good companies, what to look for in a hospice nurse, and how to get things going. Although hospital protocol prohibited them from favoring one company over another, they gave me the names of a couple well-respected options and I went with one. With that, they went off to make the phone calls necessary to kick-start the care, making sure a hospice staff person would visit our home that very night.

Logistics done, Karen and I walked to the elevator bank, dropping down two levels, out to our car, and home. Karen would never see the Huntsman Cancer Hospital again.

*****

I had arranged for Bev, one of Karen's Biola college roommates, to fly in late that afternoon from Southern California. Amber picked her up from the airport and brought her to our home. It was wintertime in Utah – dark early and cold – so Bev's arrival was a bright light, the best gift I could have imagined for the Swan family at this critical fork in the road. Her presence also gave me time to call Ryan, Allene, and Neil and explain that their mother's cancer treatment journey was over. She was now in hospice.

The hospice nurse, a younger woman, came by that evening, gathering information from me about Karen's diagnosis, treatment history, medications, and the all-important feeding tube. She stressed that hospice is all about a patient's daily comfort as much as possible. Occasionally patients go into hospice, and then back to a treatment regimen. This was unlikely to happen with Karen, principally due to the melanoma cancer in her brain and complications caused by the seizure.

We discussed logistics: who to call in an emergency; how medications would be ordered; and how often the hospice nurses would come to the house to check on Karen's condition. In some ways, it was an odd, uncomfortable conversation; the elephant in the room was that in a matter of weeks, Karen could die, in this very house. Whether that occurred in weeks or months was not for us to know.

This "new, new normal," called hospice was another chance to live one day at a time. We had never been on this road before, and there were many unknowns. Fortunately, friends like Bev sat with Karen in the living room for hours, using creative workarounds to communicate. On sunny days, I would disconnect the pump, bundle Karen up, and these long-time friends would go on slow, meandering walks in the neighborhood.

As with Gail Kopetz earlier in the month, Karen and I brought Bev to the Planetarium to see Karen's favorite movie, Jerusalem. Once again, this hour-long IMAX film had the same powerful effect on her spirit, as she pounded her chest at several points, and wept at the end.

Not only did Bev serve Karen, she served me, including making delicious meals every night of the week, encouraging me as I made one decision after another, and when Amber dropped by, loving her as she would her own daughter, as only a mother knows how.

Amber, fiercely loyal to her mother, gave of herself in exemplary ways, even as she worked two jobs and lived thirty minutes away. She would drive over after one of her jobs, bathe and/or wash Karen's hair, do Karen's nails, take her on short walks, play her violin while Karen soaked it all in, or just sit next to her mom, caressing her, holding her hand. Amber seemed to realize that every moment was valuable and precious, and there is no doubt in my mind that she was given extraordinary strength to jam 25 hours of stuff into a 24-hour day. If she could be there, she was there.

It was love in action.

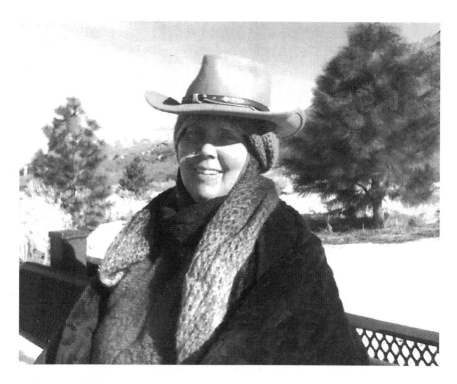

Karen at a park in Sandy – January 2014

-32-

Making a Family Memory

First California Week

Towards the end of January 2014, Karen and I had some horribly difficult but necessary discussions: Where she wanted to spend her last days, Utah, or Vista, CA?

She chose Vista.

I called her parents, Chet and Marjorie Scheltema, and asked whether they would be willing to host Karen and I in their home, and how they would feel about their daughter spending her last days there. I gave them the details about Karen entering hospice, her daily routine, what might happen in the weeks ahead, and told them to think about the decision. A day later, they called me back. To their great credit, they were willing to swallow that potentially bitter pill – that their daughter might die in their home – and invited us to move down.

After discussing Karen's wishes with our children, on a snowy January 31 morning, Karen, Bev and I piled ourselves, Bev's suitcase, Karen's meds, the feeding pump, cases of nutrient, and a ragtag assembly of Karen's and my clothing items into a car and started off for California, 720 miles away. I drove; Karen sat in the front right seat, and Bev, in the rear, keeping an eye on both Karen and the all-important nutrient pump, now running on internal batteries.

Stops were frequent, as nutrient and water quickly filled Karen's bladder. Because I kept Karen somewhat sedated with regular doses of Lorazepam, Bev and I walked Karen into convenience-mart restrooms, arm-in-arm, trying to maintain her dignity by not drawing too much attention. When Karen was more alert, we would listen to music, talk, or watch the landscape slowly change from snowy mountains to open desert.

*****

5 p.m.

We stopped in Vegas for the night. Bev had a room by herself. I set up Karen's and my room like it was our master bedroom at home: pole stand for the water and nutrient bags; meds, measuring spoons and cups carefully laid out on the counter; and syringes of various sizes awaiting the medication infusion schedule that we needed to keep.

Exhausted from the 350-mile drive, I quickly changed Karen's cloths and tucked her into bed. Within seconds, she was drifting off to sleep. Strange, I know, but I viewed that as a gift; it gave me time to prepare for the long evening ahead before I, too, crashed from fatigue.

I followed my normal routine throughout the night, which included checking Karen's feeding tube to make sure it had not pulled out, squeezing her meds – in the rights doses – through the tube, and listening to her breathing quietly, indicating that the Lorazepam was still working its magic.

It was a tough night, but we made it. Next morning, Bev helped me pack everything up, move the stuff to the car, eat a quick breakfast provided by the hotel, and walk Karen down to the lobby. A six-hour drive down I-15 lay ahead of us. Destination: Vista.

We arrived at Karen's folk's home after dusk, tired but safe. Probably most important, the feeding tube stayed in its place. In addition, I knew there were dozens and dozens of moving parts to make this two-day trip even remotely possible, and it had been a success, certainly way beyond my expectations or cleverness.

Clearly, Someone was watching over us, protecting us.

Karen's folks had prepared their home for our arrival, showing a helpfulness that told me they took their first-born child's illness very seriously. Even so, it had been five months since they last saw their daughter, and during that time she had lost the ability to talk, there was a tube coming out of one of her nostrils, and she needed help walking into their home. The vibrant woman they had seen come bounding through the door in past visits was no more.

Two days, 720 miles plus many, many bathroom stops meant an exhausted Karen. While Bev and Karen's father unloaded the car, Karen's mother and I prepared Karen for bed, going through my nightly routine with Marjorie at my side. Normally, I would sit next to Karen until she fell asleep. Now that we were with her folks, I invited one of them to sit with her, and to either quietly talk to her, read some passages from the Bible, or simply pray silently for her. Both on this night and in the ones ahead, her folks jumped at the chance to spend this time with their daughter.

Later that night, Bev's husband, Darrel, arrived to bring her back home to the L.A. area. That was the last time they would see Karen. Like Rose, Gail, Joan, Bernadette and many others, Bev's tangible love for my family was love lived out.

The daily routine I had set up for Karen in Utah did not change much, except that Karen's mother, a retired nurse, helped me with tasks big and small, like Karen using the toilet, showering, getting ready for bed, or reading to her when she was in bed. Often, her father sat next to his daughter in the living room or our bedroom, just to keep her company.

Like in Utah, Karen enjoyed sitting in the living room, whether it was upright in a rocking chair, snuggled under some blankets lying on a sofa, or falling asleep with her head on my shoulder. We had no doctors to visit anymore, no house to take care of. My mother-in-law fixed me delicious meals, a welcome change from my limited, functional food habits. The nutrient pump was a constant companion, as was the medication cycle. Essentially, Karen and I just settled in.

I arranged for staff from a new hospice company to come to our "adopted" home and assess Karen. They showed up the day after we arrived, evaluating Karen's physical and emotional state, and obtaining detailed medicine dosing information from me. I had also arranged for a huge shipment of nutrition cans, bags, and syringes, enough to cover us for a couple months. Better to have too much than not enough.

Karen had two sisters in the Southern California area, Rose, and Coral, and family dynamics between them, Karen, and the parents made for some challenges, at least initially. Karen was closest to Rose by far. Rose and her daughter drove from their home three hours north to spend a day, mid-week, with Karen, mainly just to "hang out."

Understandably, Coral also wanted to see her dying sister. One day Rose and Coral wound up at the house at the same time. Although everyone was polite, wiser from that experience, I arranged for them to come at separate times, creating some boundaries. Resolution of long-simmering issue would have to occur another time, if at all.

Families are complicated. Assuming positive intent, I would say that everyone in Karen's family was just trying to do the best they could in the midst of some very trying circumstances.

One day blurred into the next, mostly time spent around the Vista home. Other than the hospice nurse's daily monitoring visit, it was just Karen, her folks, and I. Occasionally I would disconnect Karen from the pump and we would go on a very short walk.

A favorite memory was the mid-week day I put her in the car and we drove down to one of her favorite coastline overlooks. It was an overcast February day, but her eyes brightened when she saw the ocean waves, surfers, birds, sailboats, and best of all, sunset. Like old times, out came the point-and-shoot camera; Karen fired off a couple of photos, classics that showed that her keen, artistic eye was still working.

Mid-week, fatigue almost got the best of me. I sent a text to my four children, suggesting that perhaps the upcoming Week 2 was not such a good idea after all. Maybe we should call it off and drive Karen back to Utah? To their credit, all my children immediately responded, alarmed yet firm, telling me that we should stay the course; time as a family on the beach was important, and they would help me with the various tasks that were wearing me down. With that exhortation, I pushed through the next few days, awaiting their arrival.

Towards the end of the Vista week, we began a slow-motion transition to Week 2 of our stay in California. Our children were gathering from distant spots; the six Swans would soon be together once again.

*****

<u>Second California Week</u>

From his residence way up in Alaska, Ryan had seized the initiative, renting a furnished guesthouse via the Internet, located right on the beach in Oceanside, California, not more than fifteen minutes from my in-laws' home. It had two bedrooms, kitchen and expansive family room on the main floor, with large windows that gave us an unobstructed view of the Pacific. In addition, there was another bedroom, kitchenette, and bathroom on the lower floor.

Our February occupancy meant low season, with tourists walking along the beach.

On Saturday morning, Allene flew into SoCal from Oregon, Amber and Neil from Utah, and Ryan, Alaska. Because of logistics, they flew into a variety of Southern California-area airports, and friends, including my long-time friend, Rod, helped transport them to Oceanside. Fortunately, Rod, who had been so instrumental in supporting me over the years, dropped Neil off at my in-laws' home and was able to see Karen.

My children had come up with the guesthouse idea; in happier times it would have been a wonderful place for a family vacation. This was different. We had gathered to spend time together because Karen was dying, and unless something dramatic happened, the six of us would not likely be together again.

So, sandwiched in between Karen's daily nutrient, medication, and sleeping routine, my children pulled together to go the local supermarket and prepare all the meals. In addition, at least one person was either sitting with Karen on the couch while she was awake, next to her as she looked out the picture windows facing the ocean, or holding her hand as she slept on that same couch. Then there were her normal toilet and shower needs; my children really stepped up to the plate with these tasks.

Most memorable were the many times we would gather outside, in front of the house, sitting together on beach chairs on the sand, enjoying the sun's warmth, the setting sun, swimming performances of dolphin pods moving up and down the coast just offshore, and drinking in the smells and sounds of the water hitting the sand. Ryan made campfires every night.

Since Karen could still walk, it was not uncommon for one or two of her children to walk beside her down to the water or along the beach for a few yards. Karen loved the ocean and bred this love into her children. It was a rich, memorable, indescribable time when we were together outside.

As this was a Swan family gathering, I severely limited the number of visitors who could come by, making sure my children were in full agreement before giving the green light to guests. My dear sister, Colleen, drove down from L.A. and spent a day with us. Rose came down another day, bringing some homemade meals for us to use in the days ahead. The only other visitors were the hospice nurse, and one day, a social worker. The latter person attempted to help the six of us process the strong emotions we were feeling about Karen's decline, and grievances some of my children had about my hesitations regarding the beach house plan.

Unfortunately, none of us knew the social worker; she had parachuted into our presence unaware of our history or the specific feelings we were facing. Other than me offering a heartfelt apology to my children while she was there, on hindsight, bringing her into our gathering was probably a mistake. It was a very hard day for me; I felt like a failure.

I attempted to have a pastor from my in-laws' church come to pray with the family, but again, none of the children knew him and most were not interested in a well-meaning stranger bringing religious words into our setting. I got it.

To everyone's credit, we did our best to show patience and love towards one another during that brief, intense week. We created some lasting memories together, even if it will take some time to process them. Pictures taken that week help tell the tale.

In the evenings, several of my children helped me walk Karen down the stairs to our room on the bottom floor. Once there, my daughters and I would begin the familiar routine of getting her changed, swapping out her nutrient bags, lining up her meds for the next twelve hours, and then winding her down for the night, where ideally, she would quickly fall asleep. Once asleep, one of my children would sit with their mother while I took a break.

Although we were in the same house, the two levels, especially at night, made the downstairs room feel detached from social interactions on the top floor. To address this, towards the end of the week we experimented with having Karen sleep in one of the bedrooms upstairs. While neither option was ideal, having Karen upstairs round-the-clock cut down on the upstairs-downstairs logistics and seemed to increase our connections with each other.

*****

One night, as Karen and my children relaxed in the top floor family room, I headed downstairs to call my long time friends and Christian counselors, Ken and Mary, who lived in Fresno, California. I had slipped into some depression after the recent session with my family and the social worker, so emotionally and physically spent that I did not know if I could go on.

Ken and Mary were there for me at that very desperate time; they carefully listened and praised me for what I had done to serve Karen, in the midst of some very intense family time. While they knew that I wasn't looking for vindication, they also knew that I just needed to hear that I wasn't a complete failure.

Their words that night, on the phone, in my darkened lower-floor room, were a balm to my bruised spirit. "This, too, shall pass," I recall Ken saying. He was right. As the conversation wound down, they prayed for Karen, my children, and I.

That phone call was one of the most significant conversations I had with anyone during the seven-year cancer journey. The compassion and understanding those two friends showed me at a very critical time made a huge difference in my life. While I felt completely alone in the world, on a small island all by myself, they joined me, simply to be with me, to love me.

Our "beach house" days flew by surprisingly fast, and since checkout was Friday morning, a critical decision loomed just a few days ahead. Did Karen want to stay in Vista, or return to Sandy? As Karen and I snuggling together on the couch on a beautiful Thursday morning, I leaned over to her and asked the question: Vista, or Sandy?

She mouthed, Sandy.

That seemed right. On hindsight, Karen needed this trip to Vista for closure with her childhood home, her folks, and her beloved ocean. That goal met, and as the clock continued ticking down, her heart drew her back to Sandy, her home since 1990. There was no wavering or indecision on her part.

Suddenly, the five of us had a task; get the house ready for our departure and all the logistics planned for the six of us heading three different directions the next day. Thursday become a carefully choreographed team effort to keep Karen comfortable, as my children and I packed, cleaned, and lined everything up to head out early the next morning. Four of us would drive back to SLC in a large rented SUV, while Allene flew to Boise and Neil to Salt Lake. There were a lot of moving parts; my children stepped up, doing an extraordinary job.

*****

Friday

We said our good-byes to Allene and Neil, and then Ryan, Amber, Karen, and I headed over to Vista to see Karen's folks, thinking this might be the last time they would see their daughter alive. It was a short, pensive time; each of Karen's parents came to the open passenger car door and hugged Karen, lingering by her. Any spoken words were private. As events would play out in the weeks ahead, this would be the last time Karen's father saw her alive.

Ryan was at the wheel of the SUV as we hopped on I-15 northbound, our vehicle jammed packed with people, suitcases, emotions, and a dozen cases of nutrient that had been shipped to us two weeks earlier. It would be a 720-mile mad dash to Salt Lake, all in one day; Karen was getting weaker and we needed to get her back to the comfort of her own home. We had driven this route many, many times before, albeit in happier days. This time, we simply did what we had to do.

Like our trip south from Salt Lake City two weeks ago, I kept Karen on her feeding pump and medication schedule the entire way home. After three months of practice, it was a familiar routine, made more challenging because, well, we were on a long road trip. Nutrient, water, and medications – chilled and at room temp – were managed at rest stops and McDonald's parking lots. My vital goal and prayer: keep germs out of Karen's feeding tube. Thankfully, with Ryan and Amber's assistance, we pulled it off.

The more practical challenge was bathroom stops. Even though Karen was wearing an adult diaper, because of her purely liquid diet, plus the constant infusion of water, those would easily soak through. That meant that around every thirty minutes, Amber or I would ask Karen if she needed to use the restroom. She used hand signals to respond.

Toilet breaks, rather routine in normal life circumstances, were especially tough, because since I gave Karen Lorazepam to keep her comfortable and calm, the result was that she could barely walk. Consequently, two of us would slowly, carefully glide Karen out of the SUV and walk/carry her into a crazy, crowded, marginally sanitary public restroom areas (fast food place, convenience mart, highway rest area, etc.). Reaching the female restroom, Amber took over; maneuvering her mom into a stall, making sure she did not fall over along the way. Once there, she helped Karen with the toilet, washed two sets of hands, and then reversed course out to Ryan and I, waiting to guide Karen back to the car. Off we would go, until the next stop.

*****

Since my insurance plan would not cover interstate hospice companies, I had to recruit another Utah agency to assume Karen's care. I made this happen, via cell phone, while we drove north out of SoCal.

Like so many times before, there was divine intervention on this day, this time with a phone call. The last month had taught me that an experienced, compassionate, responsive nurse is the critical link in end-of-life hospice care. I decided to use the same hospice agency that we had before leaving Utah two weeks ago, but this time, I had laser-like focus.

When I made the call, I immediately asked to speak with a supervisor. Once connected, I explained precisely what I wanted, and when: the "what" was a veteran nurse, ready to roll; the "when" was tomorrow, Saturday.

Could she make that happen?

She could.

"I recommend Camile," was the supervisor's response, "an experienced, middle-aged hospice nurse who just rejoined the agency after a sabbatical." I pressed her for details on this woman because we could not afford to have a new, unresponsive or annoying hospice nurse show up the next day. Satisfied with what I heard, I asked that Camile call me, which she did within the hour, and I "interviewed" her as we cruised along at 80 mph.

Just by talking with her on the phone, I knew Camile was the one, a Godsend. I explained the situation, including that we were on the road driving out of California for Utah. Could she come to our Sandy home tomorrow?

"Are you sure you want me to come tomorrow?"

"Yes! Absolutely."

She was all in. "I will be there late tomorrow morning."

That done, I made one more call, to Blue Cross, confirming that hospice care coverage would restart tomorrow in Utah and that they would cover it. They would.

Ryan drove the entire 720 miles from Vista to Sandy, an impressive effort in itself, getting us home mid-evening. It had been a long, safe, successful trip. Karen was now in <u>her</u> home, where she wanted to be. The first priority was to warm up the house and get her in bed. Amber knew the steps by heart, helping me with her mom as Ryan unloaded the SUV.

Pajamas on? Check.

Nutrient and water bags full? Done.

Meds infused? Complete.

Electric blanket on and bed warm? Felt good!

Amber and I tucked Karen into bed; she fell asleep almost immediately.

Ryan, Amber, and I were not far behind.

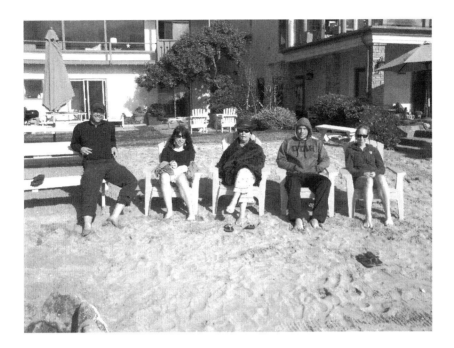

Ryan, Allene, Karen, Neil, Amber – Oceanside, CA

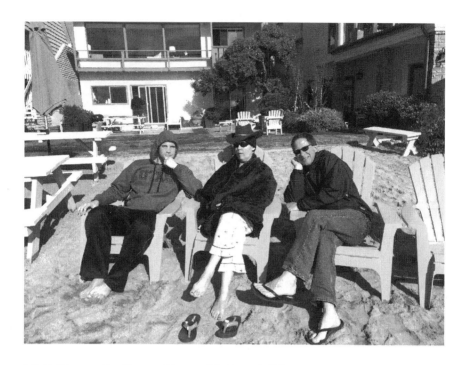

Neil, Karen, Sterling – Oceanside Beach House

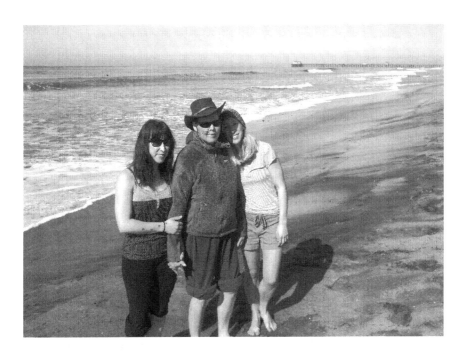

Allene, Karen, Amber – Oceanside Beach House

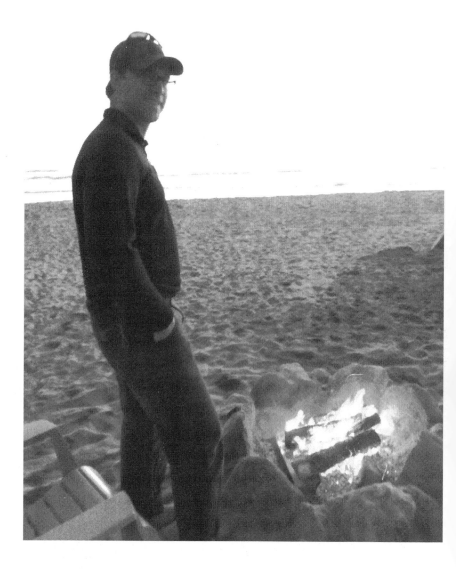

Ryan – Oceanside beach house

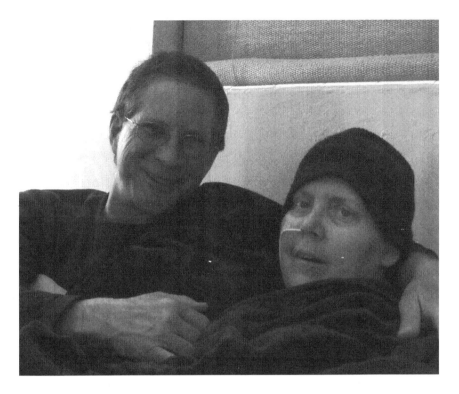

Sterling, Karen – Beach House – February 2014

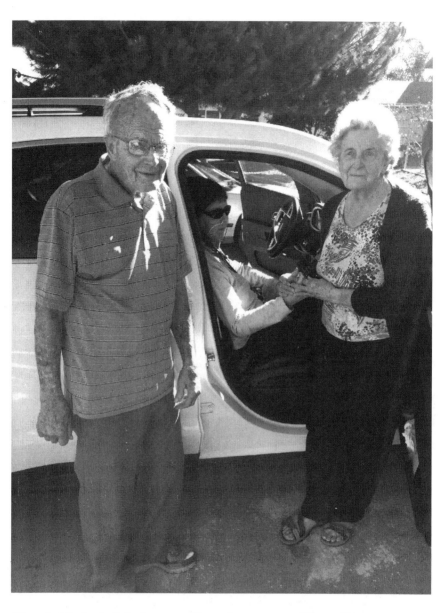

Chet & Marjorie Scheltema – Karen's parents – Vista, CA

~33~

Hospice

As promised, Camile was at our door late morning. After watching her interact with my wife for only five minutes, I knew she was the right person. Most importantly, Karen warmed to her, as did Amber, not an easy one to impress. Even during this first visit, Camile calmly provided me essential guidance for this last chapter of Karen's journey. The California experience – to Vista, then Oceanside – was over. Karen would not be returning to the Huntsman, either. As the face of the hospice agency, Camile was now our guide, doing what she humanly could to serve Karen and keep the Swan boat from tipping over.

Following Camile's assessment of Karen, and dozens of questions & answers going back and forth between the two of us, we agreed that she would initially come daily to get a baseline on Karen's overall trends, build trust with her, and help me manage any medication changes or complications. Although Camile was not there to "heal" Karen, her responsiveness gave me hope that I could deal with events in the days ahead, even though I had no idea what was coming.

Glad I didn't.

*****

While Amber returned to work and her home close to downtown Salt Lake, Ryan remained in the Sandy area for a few more days, staying with friends at night but coming over each day to spend time with his mom in the living room. I saw it as a unique time for mother and first-born child together, never to be repeated.

Friday morning came, and with that, a knock at the door. A friend of Ryan's was there ready to take him to the airport, where he would fly back to Alaska. In my mind's eye, I still see Ryan giving Karen a sustained hug, and I can still feel the hug he gave me. With that, he was off. It would be the last time he saw his mother alive, at least in person.

"Time to call out the cavalry; all hands on deck," said Camile to me one day as I walked with her out to her car. "Time to use every family member and friend IOU you ever saved. You are going to need help, Sterling. Don't be proud. Ask for help. Do it now!"

Really? What was so urgent? I had managed for seven years. Yes, things might have been a bit crazy at times, but we survived. Why did I need to call in IOU's all the sudden?

Camile saw storm clouds on the horizon, and since I had given her permission to help me navigate the path ahead, she was doing just that.

Within the hour, I was on the phone with Karen's sister, Rose. "Can you come for another week, Rose? The hospice nurse told me to call in all my IOU's, and you were the first one to come to mind."

Rose said she would.

Until she showed up, Amber squeezed even more minutes out of her already-full days to come over and spend time with her mom (bathing, hair, fingernails, violin concertos, reading, touching, etc.), which allowed me time to run errands or spend a few minutes with Jeff Nellermoe, my pastor friend.

As Jeff transitioned away from his local church pastoral responsibilities, he had more and more time to spend with me. I had grown up in church settings, so I knew it was extremely rare for pastors to have spontaneous time available on their schedules. He did. Plenty.

These February and March months proved unique for both Jeff and I. Typically, I would text him when I had a few minutes free, asking to meet me at Starbucks. Often I would hear back almost immediately: Yes, let's do it now; or, yes, how about in an hour? When I couldn't find a way to get out of the house, Jeff would come to me.

Often, he pulled up in front of my house, two cups of coffee in the cup holders, and we would talk about how I should plan for Karen's impending death.

- The Memorial Service
- Burial options
- My children's possible reactions

- Extended family issues
- My own fatigue and confusion

Equally valuable, he regularly prayed with me for my family and I, even if I did not know how or for what to pray. Much more than "happy talk" or therapy, these prayers had power; many were answered way beyond my human expectations. Jeff was Providentially "dropped" into my life scarcely two months prior to Camile's "all hands on deck" urging, a presence that would sustain me during some very turbulent weeks ahead.

Neil, although living on the University of Utah campus and carrying a full load of science-related classes, came by the house whenever possible. He was a bright light filling our home; sometimes bringing a dog, other times, a Ukulele. It did not take much to bring Karen joy these days; one could tell she felt things deeply when she pounded on her chest.

Then there were Karen's long-term friends, those who were not afraid of cancer or mortality, and canceled other things to be with my wife. Some showed up at the door, impromptu; others called first, saying they wanted to drop by. Either approach was fine. Karen saw me a lot. What she and I both needed were her girlfriends to come by and shower her with love.

Since the news had spread that Karen was in hospice, I was once again frequently asked the question: What can I do? I gave the same answer, year-in, year out. Be there! Show up! It was that simple.

People did not have to bring food (although I would gladly take that), material gifts, or promise to come "when things slowed down." They just had to come, for five minutes or a half hour. There were a handful of Karen's friends and family that "got" this basic principle; most others missed the window of opportunity, so when Karen started her rapid decline, it was too late. During her final days, I was severely limiting visitors.

To the astonishment of our friends out-of-state, many of our past and present neighbors, religious or not, male or female, did some of the "heavy lifting" for Karen and I during January through March. For example, Jack, a past neighbor, stopped by our home whenever he was in the area bidding on remodeling projects. If our door was open, he stopped and knocked, bringing energy and laughter in with him.

Our current neighbors were simply amazing. Meals came regularly. Wives would sit with Karen while I ran errands. Husbands would come over and offer to hang out with me. These things happened so often that I thought it was normal, only to have people tell me later how exceptional this concern was in our busy, impersonal world. These neighbors, friends all, surrounded Karen, my children, and I, in some profound and deeply meaningful ways. The little things became the big things.

Last but not least, a friend from my FAA days and his wife drove an hour to see Karen and I, delivering a blanket, praying for us, and spreading joy all around. As the three of us stood in the driveway before they left, Matt made a comment about how supernatural things often occur when a person is dying, and that I should pay attention. His words proved prophetic.

*****

In late February I was at my dentist's office for a check-up, a familiar spot for my family for over two decades. Dr. Matt Webb and his staff knew about Karen's cancer and clearly cared. On that day, as he always did, Dr. Webb asked how Karen was doing. I described the difficulty of brushing her teeth, explaining that the best I could do was use a warm face cloth saturated with mouthwash to gently rub her teeth, mouth, and tongue.

He thought for a moment and then asked if I would be willing to bring her in during their lunch hour when there were no other patients in the office. He promised to carefully clean her teeth using every trick in his dentist toolbox. I pitched this offer to Karen, and characteristically, she said yes.

A couple days later, Karen found herself in a dental chair. Dr. Webb and one of his senior dental assistants manually rubbed all of her teeth with small, lightly abrasive tissues, carefully sucking any liquid out of her mouth. I sat over in a corner, watching. What I saw was love in action. Over a period of what seemed an hour, they treated Karen with the utmost care and respect. Alone with my thoughts, I could barely hold back my tears.

Once done, Karen stood up from the exam chair, and as she did, I watched in wonder as Dr. Webb, followed by staff, gave

Karen sustained hugs. It was the closing of another chapter; none of them would ever see her again. A month later, Dr. Webb took time off from his practice to attend Karen's funeral.

Encountering these types of folks along the cancer journey strengthened my faith in humanity. I met dozens and dozens of them in every walk of life.

Dr. Webb, to you and your staff, thank you.

*****

Starting in late February, Karen's day began around 6 a.m. Most of time she wanted a shower to warm up. After that, I would get her dressed, and then together we would walk into the living room and over to "her" recliner chair. Surrounded by layers of blankets and pillows, she settled in, watching the sunrise, our neighborhood come alive, and occupying herself with crafts, music, or light reading. A new round of nutrient, water, and meds came next. Then, I ate breakfast. Once all this was done, we waited for the day to play itself out.

When Karen had to use the restroom, ideally there were two family members or friends walking with her, one person steadying her so she would not fall, another rolling the stand carrying the pump, nutrient, and water. Getting the fifty feet to the restroom required some teamwork; everyone played a part, including Karen. As her stability declined, walking was out; rolling was in, using a four-wheeled walker equipped with a seat.

Pushing her fast, but not too much, was fun for everyone. Even with the balance issues, Karen was still strong. It was not uncommon for her to grab the door molding as we exited the bathroom and hold on. I never figured out whether this clutching was because she was being silly, hesitant, or something else. No matter. I would lay my hand over hers, carefully prying the fingers off the molding one at a time. Free at last, off in the walker we'd go, accelerating into the living room until the last second.

Towards the end of February, Camile arranged for Dr. Anna Beck, an oncologist with the hospice agency and Huntsman Cancer Hospital, to come to our home for an assessment of Karen's condition. On the day of her visit, Amber was there, too. At one point, as Amber and Camile walked Karen to the restroom, I watched Dr. Beck observing Karen's gait and balance. That led to a brief, private discussion between us about her nutrition, its value, volume, and when to stop the feeding. It was a candid, important, and very sobering five minutes.

Dr. Beck recommended minimal visual stimulation (i.e., TV), since Karen's brain was already stressed enough. In addition, as her decline accelerated, the oncologist explained that Karen would sleep more, even during the day. Finally, I was reminded again that when a cancer patient gets to this point, the body wants to die. It was the natural course of things.

Natural or otherwise, Dr. Beck's comments made me want to throw up. The thought of Karen dying seemed so unimaginable. Yet, like so many times before, I remembered my caregiver role, at times a miserable job, and pressed ahead. Her message was clear. Absent a dramatic turn-around, Karen would soon die.

*****

In the midst of this heavy discussion, two 1,000-pound gifts arrived! Mim Nellermoe and a teenage friend came riding up on a pair of horses, right into our front yard. Dismounting, Mim brought Maxi, her treasured Arabian, close to the front windows so Karen could spot this magnificent horse.

That was enough!

Up sprung Karen; she was going out.

So were the rest of us.

We maneuvered the walker outside so Karen could sit down while interacting with Mim, Amber and the horses. It was a magical, powerful time, including when Amber hopped up on Maxi, Karen's favorite.

Dr. Beck and Camile spent about 15 minutes outside, admiring the horses with the rest of us, and in particular, interacting with Karen. Both were class acts.

They soon departed, as did the cowgirls. It had been a bittersweet afternoon, starting with serious words, concluding with friends riding animals that, to Karen and Amber, represented pure joy. Did angels ride on horses? On this day, they did.

*****

Apart from this brief adventure, Karen showed little interest in going outside, even to stand on the steps and watch the sunset. The Outdoor Woman was starting to pull inside. Changes were accelerating.

Increasingly, Camile and I began chasing symptoms and side effects in Karen, such as sleep deprivation, constipation due to the nutrient, congestion due to a cold, and decline in her ability to express her needs through writing. Weekdays, I could count on Camile showing up to help me strategize around these and other issues; on weekends, I was left to call the Hospice Nurse Line.

Nurses-on-call is a blessing and a curse. On the up side, they could help with urgent needs, such as brainstorming solutions to an acute problem; on the downside, it often took a while for these on-call nurses to get to the house. More importantly, although they were generally competent, they were not Camile, nor did they understand Karen's history.

This left me in a role reversal. When they walked through the door, I got the on-call nurse quickly up to speed on what was going on with Karen, and would often suggest solutions to the problem at hand.

The pressing problem was worsening congestion in Karen's sinuses and lungs. Camile, the on-call nurses, and I spent most of our time together brainstorming possible short-term answers to this critical condition, such as trying a different decongestant, more frequent showers, or when all else failed, a bulb syringe.

Since there was no effective way of sucking all that mucus out of Karen's sinuses and lungs, minus a magic wand for making everything dry up and disappear, I reverted to an old-fashioned technique, cleaning out her nasal passages with Q-tips and a bulb syringe. It was the best I could do with a bad situation.

Ten years earlier, I would have never done this. Now, learning to love, I was willing to do so. Serving Karen was changing my life, one choice at a time.

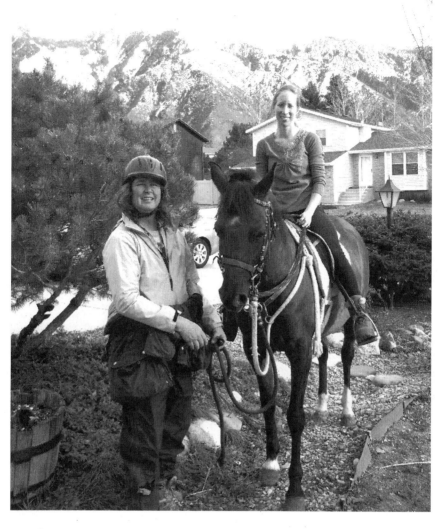
Mim Nellermoe, Amber

~34~

Decline – Part 1

Before she left my home earlier in the week, Dr. Beck gave me a few key words of advice, echoing almost exactly those Dr. Grossmann had prophetically expressed six weeks earlier: immediately start tapering Karen off her nutrient, from the 2,000 calories/day she had been receiving since Thanksgiving, stepping down through 1500, 1200, and stopping at 600 calories/day over the next three days. Specifically, I should feed Karen in the morning at the normal pump rate, and when I had reached the targeted calorie number for that day, stop. Water throughout the day was fine, but no more food until the next morning.

I could barely wrap my head around this recommendation? Drop Karen to 600 calories/day in three days? After all, that's the calorie count of a couple of slices of pizza or a large hamburger. Up to this point, I had moved mountains to make sure Karen received around 2,000 calories/day, even when we were out on a walk, viewing an IMAX movie, or driving to California. Now, I was going to consciously decrease her food intake, dramatically so?

Camile agreed with Dr. Beck. The time had come to take this hard step.

I discussed the taper recommendation with Karen.

Somehow she knew the stakes and willingly accepted it.

I delayed implementing the taper until I could talk with my sons and daughters. I didn't want them to hear second-hand that something so serious had happened without their knowing about it first. In the midst of my communication effort, something more ominous and infinitely more difficult occurred.

The next day, Camile came for Karen's daily assessment. Afterward, she asked me to walk with her out to the car. Once outside, she hit me with a bombshell message. She and Dr. Beck had talked further, agreeing that it was time for Karen to soon go off all nutrients.

Altogether?

Completely?

Yes.

They recommended I taper Karen down to 600 calories/day over the next three days, and then stop entirely.

After observing her, they concluded that Karen's body was broadcasting a loud, clear message: I am in decline. In their professional opinions, the nutrient was not making things better, only worse.

Much worse.

*****

By now, Rose had arrived from Southern California. It was good to have her back again. She knew the ropes, I trusted her, Karen had declined much further since her last visit in early January, and we were facing a crisis.

After talking personally with each of my four children and gaining their understanding (mixed with sorrow) of the taper recommendation, I began the taper, three steps, over three days, down to 600 calories/day. That was technically "easy" to do. The much bigger step – a huge leap over a Grand Canyon filled with emotion – was cutting off all nutrition, including how Karen would signal us when she wanted to stop eating completely?

Camile had a suggestion regarding this signaling issue, shared with me outside after one of her daily visits:

Step 1 – Place a can of nutrient by Karen's living room chair so it was close and in her line-of-sight

Step 2 – After drawing close to her, say, kneeling next to her chair, occasionally ask if she wanted something to eat while pointing at the can.

Step 3 – If she nodded yes, I should give her one can of nutrient, which contained about 250 calories. If she shook her head no, hold off for a couple hours and ask again.

With that, Camile left.

I pondered what she had recommended. Wrestled with the implications. Wondered if there was another way.

There was not.

Every cell in my body, every ounce of loyalty and love, screamed in me, NO, NO, NO!!

Yet…I knew what I needed to do.

Later on that day I initiated one of the most difficult conversations I have ever had with my wife, asking, "Is it time for you to stop eating entirely?" I shared with her the recommendation from Dr. Grossmann, Dr. Beck, and Camile. I explained that her body would tell her what it needed, if anything. When that point came, we would figure out a way for her to communicate with me. There was no rush. No one was trying to starve her to death. In no way was I going to persuade her to stop eating.

This was her call, on her terms, in her time.

She squeezed my hand. We hugged. She wept, as a wave of sadness hit me. While Karen could no longer write intelligible words, she understood.

*****

Saturday and Sunday, March 1 & 2

Now that I had discussed the food termination topic with Karen, I called my children to discuss this life-ending step with each of them. Should Karen decide she was ready, I wanted make sure that none of this surprised them, even if they violently reacted to the implications of the decision. While each was onboard with the taper-to-600 calories recommendation, the more radical one, suspending food entirely, took some time to process. Eventually, each of them agreed that their mom had the right to make the feeding decision, even though such a step ran counter to the basic human urge to preserve life.

When Saturday morning came, Rose and I maneuvered Karen from the master bedroom into the living room, where we settled her into her favorite chair and surrounded her with layers of blankets and soft pillows. Why layers? It was wintertime, and her body was no longer producing normal levels of heat due to the significant drop in caloric intake. Rose sat close to Karen, interacting as sisters do.

After some time had elapsed, I walked out into the kitchen, grabbed a can of nutrient and slowly moved towards Karen's recliner. Kneeling down beside her, I placed the can on a bookshelf to her right, at eye level, and pointing said, "Would you like some food?"

She nodded, yes.

I opened the can, poured the 250 liquid calories into a drip bag and started the pump. In no time the brown liquid merged with an equal amount of water, squeezed through the tube, eventually ending up in her intestines.

A few hours later, I repeated the same two steps:

Point at a full can.

Ask the question.

Each time she nodded, yes.

When Sunday came, the same was true. Each time I pointed and asked, the answer was yes.

Rose had planned on staying through early March, and suddenly, it was upon us. As the days blurred into one another, I had yet to find another family member or friend who would take the hand-off from Rose to help Karen and I. Desperate, I called Marjorie, my mother-in-law, then in her late 70's, explained that her daughter was in decline, and would she please, please fly up to help.

Alone.

Immediately.

She agreed.

She booked a flight which would bring her to Salt Lake on Tuesday, two days hence, allowing an overlap with her daughter Rose, who would fly home a day later.

*****

Monday, March 3

Like the previous two days, Rose and I got Karen up from her bed, dressed her, moved her to the living room recliner chair and wrapped her with layers of blankets. Once the three of us had settled into our "living room" routine, I knelt next to her, pointed to a can of nutrient, and asked if she wanted food.

She shook her head: No

Taken back, I looked at Rose, who looked back at me, eyes wide. Distressed.

I asked a second time.

"Do you want some food?"

Again, Karen shook her head from side to side.

I looked at Rose. Tears in her eyes, she nodded.

I got up and walked into the kitchen, my head spinning. I felt like I would fall over. Was this a nightmare? Someone please tell me this is not happening.

As Karen listened to one of her favorite music playlists, and Rose sat just a few feet from her, keeping her company, I drafted an email to Ryan, Allene, Amber, and Neil, explaining that their mother had chosen not to eat that morning.

The reactions were swift, deeply personal, and gripping. Everyone knew the implications. Each wanted details of the decision, some more than others. Amber was particularly troubled by the prospect of not feeding Karen. I have no doubt the other three were, too, but Amber lived in the area and was often over at the house, watching the feeding pump whirling away, pumping nutrient into her mother's body, keeping her alive. Feeding Karen this way was not a long-term solution, but pragmatically, it had worked for over three months.

I shared Amber's turmoil and agony. Over the last seven years, Karen had rebounded so many times before that in spite of how things appeared, perhaps she would rebound again? After all, wasn't she an exceptional responder? Certainly, we were all ready for a miracle, whether some of us believed in God at the moment or not.

I did not know how to speak to this deep turmoil in Amber's heart, as I felt profoundly conflicted myself. Then I had an idea. Email Dr. Grossmann. He had allowed us this type of direct access in crisis situations, a privilege I never abused. This indeed was a crisis.

So I typed a concise email explaining Karen's condition, her decision earlier this morning, and asked him to send a non-medical, compassionate response that I could forward to my children. Within a half-hour he had responded, with one of the most sensitive, personal, yet direct emails I have ever received from any person, much less a physician.

Essentially, he explained that Karen's body was signaling that it was time for her to go. He expressed deep empathy for how difficult this decision was to accept by my children and I. Finally, he said that Karen was showing great courage and love for her family, knowing her impairment was accelerating.

I immediately forwarded both my note to him, and his response, to my four children. Soon, Amber responded with a few brief sentences, saying that although Dr. Grossmann's personal note had been hard to read, it brought her comfort.

With that, we were potentially able to proceed…down a road that no one wanted to travel…of withholding food entirely.

One more step remained.

That Monday afternoon, Amber came over to spend time with her mom. Like other days, they immediately drew close. Amber rubbed Karen's back, washed her face with a warm cloth, and at times, they even smiled. Today, she knew the stakes were high.

The can of nutrient I had set near her that morning was still there. I pulled Amber aside and repeated what Camile had suggested, which was to let Karen choose if she wanted what was in that can or not. At any time, she could point at the can and ask her mom if she wanted food.

She understood.

I said nothing more.

At one point, I saw Amber point to the un-opened nutrient can and softly ask her beloved mom if she wanted something to eat. Karen shook her head from side to side.

No.

She wanted no food.

Getting up from the chair, her face red, tears flowing, Amber left the room to grieve.

My dear daughter stayed a couple more hours; both of us asked Karen several more times if she wanted food. The answer was consistently the same.

No.

I continued giving Karen her medications and water for hydration. Rose, Amber, and I wondered aloud if her decision about food would be the same tomorrow? We would soon see.

*****

Because of Karen's food choice, my nightly routine suddenly became less complicated. I no longer had to calculate daily nutrient volumes, just focus on her medication schedule and ensure the water bag stayed full.

For about a week before Karen's decision to stop taking food, her bowel regularity was all over the place. We rode extreme pendulum swings that are very common for people using feeding tubes; a couple of days of constipation, which Camile and I would attack with laxatives, followed by a couple day of diarrhea. Those were particularly tough times.

Why constipation? The medications, nutrient, and sedentary routine threw off the body's normal rhythm. Medical staff, using dark humor, called the brew "butt cement." Dealing with Karen's bowel irregularity was a massive challenge in itself, day and night, which is one of many reasons why we rarely left the house the last couple weeks of her life.

Tuesday, March 4

As Karen sat in her "spot" in the living room, wrapped in blankets like a newborn baby, I periodically pointed to the nutrient can and asked the same question: Do you want something to eat?

For the second day in a row, she shook her head: No.

*****

Karen's morning calm, and Rose's presence, allowed me a window of time to drive 30 minutes to the airport to pick up my mother-in-law. I chose to make the run so I could fill her in on what was going on while we were in the car together.

Once at the house, Marjorie threw herself into caring for her daughter and assisting me. For next few hours, it was particularly nice to have Karen's mother and a sister in the home, together caring for my wife.

While the nutrient can remained in Karen's plain sight, she never made any motions that told us she wanted food, this even when one of us asked her directly. I enlisted Rose and Marjorie to ask "the question," to make sure biological family members also accepted Karen's unilateral, courageous, gut-wrenching, life-ending choice. As hard as that was, Rose and Marjorie needed closure on this.

In light of Karen's no-food decision, Camile started coming to my home on a daily basis. She treated Karen with great respect, often dropping to her knees next to Karen to take vitals, kicking things off with the endearing statement, "OK, dear, let's listen to what's going on inside you."

Wednesday, March 5

Transition day. Rose was heading home. She and Karen hugged, kissed and shared lots of tears, evidence of how close they were. It was the last goodbye.

Marjorie agreed to watch Karen while I ran Rose to the airport. Her nursing background, and Karen's increased pattern of dozing through much of the morning, meant that my absence was a reasonable choice. I would be back home in about an hour.

What could go wrong?

*****

As I rolled up the freeway on-ramp that would take us to the airport, to my shock, there was bumper-to-bumper traffic as far as my eyes could see. I merged in with traffic and began the stop-n-go pace so common in urban life. We had allowed a buffer to get Rose to the airport in plenty of time; but still, this amount of traffic was unusual for Salt Lake City, especially at this time of the morning.

Suddenly a huge jet of steam exploded from my engine compartment, filling even a part of the passenger compartment, and the temperature gauge on the dash immediately started climbing towards the Red zone, signaling engine overheating. I've worked on enough cars to know that this was a serious radiator problem, a huge threat to the mechanical integrity of the engine itself.

But I did not pull over or turn off the engine. Working my way over to the far left fast lane, I kept going. As the cars ahead of me finally began accelerating, so did I, pressing on to the airport and hoping that at a higher speed, perhaps the winter air would cool the engine down.

Although I was knowingly pushing my car's engine beyond its design, I was rather desperate.

Ten miles from the airport, all the red lights on my car's dash panel simultaneously burst on, screaming one message: STOP.

A mile later, the engine killed completely. I pulled right, drifting to the freeway's shoulder, just shy of an off-ramp sloping downhill…and stopped.

I did the only thing I could do…as Rose steered, I pushed my 1987 Subaru off the freeway and into a nearby parking lot.

At that point, the situation seemed completely hopeless.

- My car crippled, perhaps fatally so
- Rose's flight departing soon
- And to top it off, my mother-in-law just called to say that Karen was awake and getting agitated.

*****

"Mark, this is Sterling."

"Well hello, Sterling. What's going on? How is Karen," replied Mark, a long-time insurance agent friend in the Salt Lake area?

"Mark, I am in a bind. Are you free?"

"Yes, actually I am in between clients. How can I help you?"

"My car broke down. I am in a parking lot off I-215. Can you come <u>right now</u>, pick up my sister-in-law and drive her to the airport?"

"I know just where you are," replied Mark, "and am on my way."

Ten minutes later, Mark pulled into the parking lot. I quickly introduced him to Rose, we transferred Rose's luggage into Mark's car, and off they went. My next move was to arrange a tow truck from AAA. While waiting for the tow, I called my favorite, locally owned auto parts store and ordered a replacement radiator.

Within 15 minutes, AAA appeared, loaded my car on a flatbed tow truck, and we were on our way back to my home. As we were enroute, the auto parts store's owner called to tell me he would personally deliver a new radiator to my home that afternoon. Mark called a few minutes later; Rose made it to the airport on time.

That evening, I installed the new radiation in my Subaru, filled the completely empty cooling system, put the key in the ignition, turned it, and…

It started right up. We were not alone. Ever.

*****

Marjorie sat with Karen in the living room for hours on end, reading or doing craft work, occasionally communicating with Karen via hand signals, or words/phrases written on the ever-present notepad. Often music played on an iPod, favorites that kept her company, encouraged her spirit, or lulled her to sleep. In between these "relaxing" moments were trips to the restroom, occasional sponge baths, and the few medicines I still gave her via the tube.

Every day, Camile monitored Karen's vitals, listened to her digestive tract with a stethoscope, and made recommendations for adjusting Karen's medication, laxative, and water intake levels. It was part art, part experience, and part science, from a woman who had been a hospice nurse for years. Karen and I both trusted Camile implicitly; she also became a confidant and guide as the days blurred into one another, and the journey, completely unfamiliar and disorienting.

Absent the nutrient regimen, Karen's nightly "winding down" pattern became somewhat easier, although no less important. We kept up with her medications, comfortable fleece pajamas, warmed-up electric blanket, multiple pillows under her head to aid in breathing, plus layers and layers of blankets all around her body. Feathers and heat comforted her!

It had been quite a day! Rose left, Marjorie arrived, my car radiator blew up, I repaired it in the driveway, and now, the gift of sleep was close at hand. Although exhausted, I sat next to Karen as she lay in bed, and we talked. Well, actually, I talked a bit and she would nod or squeeze my hand when she agreed.

On that night, words did not matter. In a mystical way, we both knew it was over. She would soon depart.

We exchanged long gazes.

She nodded; I nodded.

I sang some of her favorite songs out of an old hymnal, and as she started to drift asleep, accelerated by a dose of Lorazepam, I asked Marjorie to come into the bedroom and sit next to her daughter.

Soon, Karen was asleep.

A "normal" night was ahead of us, or so I thought.

~35~

Decline – Part 2

I awoke in the wee hours of Thursday morning. Karen was moving around, restless. She had to use the toilet, and even with the adult diaper, it was better to get her to the bathroom in light of the recent bowel complications.

I got up, went to her side of the bed and steadied her as she walked into the bathroom. After over three decades of marriage, Karen and I were quite comfortable with each other's bodies, but helping her use the toilet was still a stretch.

It was my job.

As she sat on the toilet seat, I dashed out into the kitchen to grab more Lorazepam.

Seconds later I was back. As I rounded the corner into the bathroom, I watched in shock as Karen fell from a full standing position to the linoleum floor.

Crash.

She hit hard the floor hard.

Followed by a moan.

Her tongue impairment kept her from uttering a cry or scream, but I know that the fall must have hurt.

Feelings of anguish, sadness, and desperation instantly welled up inside me, but I forced them back down, way down, as I dropped to my knees to help her. With superhuman strength that came from another source, I picked her up, maneuvered her back to the toilet, cleaned her body, and put on a new adult diaper.

Once done, we stood and walked together very slowly back to her side of the bed. There, I pulled up her pajama bottoms, laid her carefully down on the mattress, piled high the blankets and pillows…and she immediately fell asleep.

Within a few minutes, so did I.

*****

Thursday, March 6

On Thursday, Camile asked Karen how she felt about not taking any more nutrients. "Are you O.K. with this, dear?"

Karen nodded yes and gave a thumbs-up.

Wisely, she turned to Marjorie, who was sitting in the living room observing Camile's care, and asked, "Are you comfortable with Karen not taking any more food?"

It was a poignant moment. Marjorie leaned her head back slightly, paused for a few seconds, and responded, "Yes, I am. I have come to believe that, although hard, this is probably best for Karen."

It was a courageous, heartfelt answer. The temptation is always there for a family member to advocate for some medical intervention, but Marjorie knew reality when she saw it. Her firstborn child, her daughter, was dying. It was time to let her go.

As Camile and I walked out to her car that afternoon, I asked, "How long does Karen have?"

"Probably a week at best," she replied.

I explained that Allene had planned to drive down from Oregon the third week in March, two weeks away. Camile thought that would be too late.

"Allene needs to be here ASAP," was Camile's frank response, "and I would be glad to communicate that urgency to her directly."

After Camile left, I immediately called Allene, explained the conversation I had just had, and encouraged her to call Camile right away.

She did.

Next morning she was on the road; by early afternoon, she was in our Sandy home, at Karen's side. I also called Ryan, Amber, and Neil, telling them that Camile believed the end was nigh.

Occasionally, friends would stop by to visit Karen. Most often, they called or texted me first, giving me a chance to explain that Karen was in decline. She could not speak, had difficulty staying awake, was struggling with chest congestion and a cold, but welcomed companionship from people she had grown to love over the years. Faced with that stark description, some people bowed out, while others were all in.

When guests arrived at the front door, I joined them on the porch, explained what to expect, and encouraged them to sit by

Karen – hold her hand, hug her, cry with her, even pray – but not talk too much. She could only handle so much. People understood and appreciated my guidance.

Those were deeply personal visits, long-time friends coming to say goodbye to Karen. For this reason alone, hospice made sense. Marjorie and I left the living room when a friend was present, so I don't even know what was shared, other than it was love. Most would never see her again.

Camile's sense of urgency pushed me to get going on something I absolutely did not want to do, which was select a local mortuary. Pastor Jeff recommended one and I went with it, a local company that had been around for decades. While it wasn't the cheapest option, they knew their business. When Karen died, I wanted things handled right.

Why cremation? Karen wanted at least half her ashes scattered in the Pacific, from a boat she had spotted years ago docked in the Oceanside Harbor. So it would be.

My plan was to drive over to the mortuary's main office on the upcoming Monday to complete the paperwork, not knowing – how could I know – that my family and I would soon be overtaken by events way beyond our control.

*****

Friday, March 7

Friday's daylight hours came and went. Karen slept much of the day. A few friends came by to pay their respects. As bedtime rolled around, Marjorie, Allene and I got Karen settled into her new hospital-type, metal frame adjustable bed that I ordered from the hospice agency and placed right next to our king bed. Marjorie, Allene, Amber or I would get Karen transitioned for sleep, and then at least one person, often two, sat with her as she drifted off.

Once asleep, at least one family member remained next to her until I was ready for bed, usually a couple hours later. I'd crawl in the king bed and move as close to the metal-frame bed as possible, stretching my arm out to touch her body.

Karen awoke early Saturday morning, agitated. Quickly moving over to the open side of her bed, I helped her stand up. We slowly walked the ten feet into the bathroom, me holding her from behind, one hand under each armpit, as she took small steps towards the toilet. Once there, I guided her as she slowly turned and sat down in the seat. Because of the fall two nights ago, I now stood next to her each time she urinated or had a bowel movement, my left arm on her right shoulder.

Suddenly, something horrible happened.

In a flash, before I could react, Karen tipped forward and accelerated, plunging head first into a corner of our small bathroom, where sheet rock, ceramic tile, and linoleum met.

She hit those surfaces with a dull thud.

Her body crumpled.

Followed by a low, deep moan.

I wanted to scream, pull my hair out, and swear at the Universe...all in one split second.

Waves of despair washed over me. I was beside myself.

Those waves continued even as I thought that while my dear wife probably had a concussion and brain trauma from this impact, it no longer seemed to matter.

Her brain, severely stressed from years of radiation, surgeries, drugs and cancer tumors, was shutting down. It would only function for a few more days.

As in the previous night's fall, I picked Karen up to a full stand. We shuffled back to the toilet, where I cleaned her body, put on a fresh adult diaper, pulled up her pajamas, and returned her to the hospital bed ten feet away.

Soon...she was asleep.

~36~

End in Sight

Among other things, Saturday morning, March 8, meant five days had elapsed since Karen's decision to stop eating. It was a profoundly bittersweet milestone.

On one hand, she was physically weaker, more lethargic, prone to cold chills, and less focused. She spent most of the waking hours in her favorite living room chair, with a prime view of the snow-capped Wasatch mountain range and her garden. In fleece pajamas and socks, an adult diaper, beanie hat, and wrapped in several layers of blankets, including a purple one bought by her dear friend, Gail, Karen passed the time with her children, mother, me, and an occasional visitor that stopped by.

On the other hand, her GI tract was starting to stabilize, which gave us time to focus on the more immediate, life-threatening need. Her head cold was making her breathing more and more difficult, and the congestion in her lungs was more pronounced by the day.

Camile and I threw everything we could think of at this very serious infection problem, that is, minus calling 911:

- Decongestants via the feeding tube
- Oral medications that Karen heroically tried to swallow
- A variety of sitting positions
- Warm air humidifier next to her chair
- And even hot baths and showers.

Unfortunately, slowly but surely, we were losing the battle.

In contrast to Karen's obvious physical decline, her indomitable spirit was as strong as ever. By all rights, she could easily have slid into a funk, but that's not who she was. Due, I am certain, to the presence of God in her life, she seemed at peace, finding joy in small things like tinkering with little items on a table next to her chair, looked at pictures with her daughters, listened to recorded music, or dozing.

Sometimes she would pick up one of her favorite artistic tools, a simple point-and-shoot camera, and start shooting pictures on boxes, her daughters' dresses still hanging on the stairs bannister, the cat, birds at our bird feeder, snow scenes, family members, and Amber as she played her violin in the living room later that day. She was clearly seeing beyond the obvious. To this day, I wonder what those things were?

*****

There were always family members in the living room with Karen, going about our small tasks, but mainly, just being with her. Yes, melanoma was killing her, but in one very limited, rational sense, on this day at least, she was fortunate; other than complications from the nasal congestion, she was relatively pain free. On hindsight, I realize this was a gift. Many end-state cancer patients suffer severe pain, an added layer of stress not only for the patient, but family helplessly watching the loved one suffer.

Although pain was not a huge issue, communication between Karen, her family and friends, and Camile, was increasingly difficult. Up through the end of February, Karen was a texting and emailing superstar. Her fingers would fly around her cell phone's slide-out full keyboard, or the iPad's touchscreen, and soon, family and friends far and wide would respond.

Once March rolled around, some of Karen's messages increasingly contained words, or even whole sentences, of gibberish. She was completely unaware of this, because in her mind, she had spelled everything correctly. Gradually, her social media recipients started contacting me, telling me sadly that the messages they were receiving from her were no longer intelligible.

It was a hard moment when I explained to Karen that we should set her cell phone aside for "awhile," since what she wanted to say was no longer getting through to her friends. I might as well have cut off her hand. After that, her world closed in.

The world shrank more today, as written communication between Karen and the family ended. All was well when Karen could write a word or phrase on the paper, expressing what she wanted or how she felt, often with a dramatic flourish or small drawing. Over this past week, her writing went from phrases, to words, to one or two letters, resulting in an awkward guessing game between Karen and those she loved. By the end of this day, Saturday, written communication, like her speech months ago, was over. We transitioned to hand signs and grunts.

While clearly frustrated, Karen never complained, whined, or slid into a pity-party. Even in that last week, she would flash her winsome smile or quietly chuckle during a lighthearted moment.

*****

As my wife's decline accelerated, I experienced an identity crisis. Why? Over the past five days, my seven-year-long "job" had gone from making sure she had proper food, water, medicine and opportunities to live life, to water and some medicines alone. I was powerless, relegated to watching my wife die. I hated it.

All these changes added up to a different "feel" in the house on Saturday. It was though our family had transitioned to a small, narrow, less clearly lit road, one that would likely soon end.

Yet, Karen was still alive. Amazingly so! She had cancer, but cancer still did not have her. She was a human being who could walk, smile, dress sharp, comb her hair, and look beautiful, even with a tube running out of her nose.

Beautiful? Really?

Yes! Absolutely!

On this day, the last Saturday of Karen's life, Amber and Allene seized the moment (carpe diem) arranging for her favorite stylist to wash and trim her hair. Next up, a pedicure, including bright blue fingernail polish, followed by a henna design carefully, lovingly applied by Allene to both Karen's hands.

She looked strikingly gorgeous, her eyes, face, and skin all looked so inviting. It was almost like old times when we were first dating.

"Hey, Karen, you look great. How about a date?"

There was more beauty to come! Amber serenaded us with several classical music pieces on her violin that afternoon. Neil jumped in next with his new Ukulele, and Karen, always the curious musician, accepted his challenge. She took the instrument and strummed a couple of bars herself. Those were treasured moments.

Yama, our family cat, not typically a "lap sitter," had recently taken up the therapy animal role, often jumping up to Karen's living room recliner, curling up at her feet, and remaining there for hours on end. When we moved Karen into the master bedroom for a nap or the night, Yama faithfully followed, again curling up at her feet. Equally touching, he would keep a close eye on things family members and I maneuvered Karen to the bathroom, wandering in there with us, watching quietly and carefully, never taking his eyes off Karen.

How to explain this?

Who was he working for? Perhaps Aslan?

No one takes a class or reads a book on what to do when a wife, mother or daughter is dying right before one's eyes. Because of Karen's lethargy and breathing discomfort, I told most friends who called that, "No, sorry, Karen is getting too weak and we can't have any more visitors." The only non-family we had in the house was Jeff and Mim Nellermoe, who again came by to "be" with Karen: touch her; pray with her; anoint her head with oil; and comfort our whole family.

That afternoon, during her normal daily visit, I told Camile about Karen's headlong plunge into the wall the previous night. She grimaced and then said, "Karen is getting too weak. It's time for a catheter bag."

Karen and I agreed. Camile, ever the resourceful nurse, made it happen right there in the master bedroom, and with that, our trips to the toilet were largely over.

Sunday, March 9

With the sunrise came Karen's last Sunday on earth. She had slept fitfully, primarily because the nasal and chest congestion was worsening. Fortunately, regular doses of Lorazepam throughout the night had kept things from getting out of control.

Once family members and I got Karen dressed for the day and settled her into the living room chair, I went to work. Camile had encouraged me to clean out Karen's nasal passages, which was not all that much different from what Karen and I had done with our infant children years ago when they had colds. Odd, but as in previous days, that experience came right back to me. Carefully leaning Karen's head back with one hand, I used the bulb syringe in the other to suck as much mucus out of her nose as possibly. Repeat…over and over.

Yes, some fluid came out, and yes, I think there was a small psychological victory to this rudimentary procedure. Anything was worth a try if it made her even 5% more comfortable.

Amber had arranged for Judy, her exceptional violin teacher and loyal family friend, to stand-by, thinking Karen was strong enough to have a private classical music concert in our living room. In addition, Karen's cancer soul sister, Cynthia, was waiting for the word to come over and see Karen for the last time. The idea was to have one, or both, drop by in the afternoon.

Unfortunately, by late morning, I was starting to physically and emotionally unravel, which is why my gut response was to tell both of these dear friends, "No." On hindsight, the better response was yes, to both. I wish I had handed off the decision and details to other family members and allowed Judy and Cynthia to come one last time, but in the midst of high-stress events, I was barely thinking straight. As the morning hours ticked by and we drifted into the afternoon, the window of opportunity closed.

Neither friend came.

*****

Because she could not blow her nose or cough, Karen's viral cold infection had migrated into the lungs. We also believe she had aspirated liquid down into that all-important organ, slowly causing her to drown in her own fluids.

Like clockwork, Camile came by the house late Sunday afternoon. It only took a few minutes for her to assess that Karen's death was nigh. Since nights were increasingly a problem for me to manage – as Karen become more and more agitated because of the congestion – Camile directed me to start giving her morphine every four hours, and stop Keppra, the anti-seizure drug, entirely. The updated objective: Keep her comfortable, but don't postpone the inevitable.

That change simplified my pharmacist role even more, Now, I gave Karen an opioid and decongestant via her "feeding" tube every four hours. Done.

I was so torn. Was I failing Karen? I would have kept that complex food, water, and medication job up forever if it had made a difference. Alas…the drugs were no longer making a difference, none except the morphine.

As night fell and Karen lay in her hospital bed, the congestion started to spike, driving her to sit up in bed, hunch over, and gasp for breath – deep, clawing gulps – over and over again. Every muscle in her torso tensed, trying to suck in air, yet it was not enough.

What would happen?

My children, mother-in-law and I, observing this trauma, had no idea what to do.

While I could have texted Camile, another idea bubbled to the surface. What about a warm mist humidifier? It was worth a try, so I ran over to a local department store five minutes from the home, getting there right before they closed, and within a half hour a cloud of warm mist, laced with an essential oil, was starting to saturate the air around Karen's bed.

That did the trick. She calmed down and soon fell asleep. The mist, going all night, morphine every four hours, and without a doubt, the prayers of many people – seen and unseen – were some of the things that carried us through that turbulent breathing period into the next morning. To those that prayed that Sunday, thank you.

Family members took turns that evening sitting at Karen's side, even though she had fallen back asleep mid-evening. To a person, we wanted her to know that she was not alone, even if her awareness level was declining. Who knows what she heard or saw? We perceive love in many different ways, in many dimensions.

Eventually, everyone else headed off to bed: Marjorie to a room just down the hall; Allene and Amber, to a room shared downstairs; Neil, to his university dorm room; and Ryan, in Alaska.

Once in bed, I snuggled up next to Karen, placing my hand on her arm, and fell asleep. Now with the catheter in use, I only got up a couple of times that night to give Karen her morphine. Apart from this, most in the house slept, no doubt fitfully, preparation for challenges ahead the next day.

*****

Monday, March 10

This morning began like many others before it. Some of my family members helped me get Karen up, into the bathroom, dressed, and safely out into the living room, where we wrapped her entire body in a pillow and blanket cocoon. We set the humidifier on a short stool right by her chair, hoping that the warm, aromatic air would give her a few more relaxed hours of breathing during the day. Soon, Yama joined her.

With the sunrise came additional warmth, light and beauty pouring into our south-facing living room. Karen could see the snow-covered mountains to the east, feast on the tulips and other perennials starting to shoot up through the barren soil, and even laugh at the hyper-active quail racing all over the yard. Although seven days without food had made her weak, her spirits were good.

They had always been good. She was a strong, optimistic Dutch-Swede woman. My daughters rearranged the room a bit so both of them could sit by their mom, one on each side. Marjorie joined them. It was a fitting setting, grandmother, mother, and twin daughters together.

Today, time had little relevance. Moment by moment, we loved Karen as best we knew how, even as we waited.

Waiting for who knew what?

I only remember making one phone call all day, to the mortuary, to verify their staff was ready to go when death arrived. I detested making those calls, since they represented finality, at least in this world. In my experience, there is nothing that focuses one's attention as much as anticipating the death of a loved one, especially a spouse or child.

As agreed, Camile came by the house late morning, warmly greeted everyone in the room, and then turned her complete attention to Karen. As she did, I told her about Karen's struggle with breathing the previous night, of running to the department store to get a humidifier, and how that helped calm things down so everyone could sleep.

Update complete, as was her habit, Camile got down on both knees, right next to Karen, adjusted her stethoscope and said to Karen, "Let's hear what's going on in there, dear." It was a tender time between Camile and Karen as she moved the stethoscope to various parts of Karen's body.

A bit of positive news: Karen's vitals and GI tract were good. The bad news: her lung congestion was only getting worse. Minus rushing Karen back into treatment, the only tools we had to combat this congestion were the decongestants, morphine, and humidifier already in use. Camile asked me how much decongestant

Karen was receiving and told me to increase it starting with the next dose.

Her daily exam complete, Camile gave Karen a hug and motioned me outside.

"I think she only has a day or two left," said Camile as we stood in the driveway.

"I am the on-call nurse tonight and only live five minutes from here. If something comes up this afternoon, this evening, or tonight, bypass the answering service and call or text me directly. I will have the phone by my bed and will immediately answer."

"This will be hard, Sterling. Hang in there."

With that, she was gone.

*****

Hospice is about choosing to die in one's own home; of hospice staff working with family to help the patient feel as comfortable as possible; and of no more interventions by physicians to address medical problems. It takes a courageous person to choose hospice, a strong commitment by the family to support the person as they decline, and an exceptional hospice nurse to keep things from falling apart.

After Camile left, Karen fell back into a light slumber. She had labored but stable breathing. When awake, she occasionally flashed her beautiful smile and waved her hand slightly to family, and those few friends who were impulsive enough to come by and bring comfort to us. Hugs and tears flowed freely.

Morning transitioned into afternoon. During her waking minutes, at least one family member, often more, would sit close to Karen, holding her hands or rubbing her back. I read very short sections of the Bible to her, the source of her strength and faith since she was a young child. Once in awhile, she would ask for a song or two from her iTunes playlist. Overall, time stood still.

Once late afternoon rolled around, we moved Karen to the master bedroom. It was much earlier than normal, but she was ready; now sleeping almost constantly, she needed something more comfortable than the recliner. Yama, glued to Karen's feet as she laid on the recliner, followed her from the living room to the master bedroom. Once we got Karen settled in the hospital bed, he settled in, too, in a tight ball at her feet.

Did he know something we didn't?

Perhaps so.

Camile had instructed me to give Karen morphine every two hours. That is a heavy dose; Karen's increasing congestion condition required serious measures. Even without a stethoscope, by leaning in close to Karen's chest, I could hear liquid in her lungs as she reflexively breathed deeply to keep herself alive. Fortunately, the morphine helped relax her, even as she was entering the last hours of life.

Night fell.

Tucked into her hospital bed and constantly surrounded by her children and mother, Karen dozed. Warm, moist air created by the humidifier calmed her a bit, as did the music playing in the next room. The lights were kept low.

We all waited.

Watched.

Any thoughts were mostly kept to ourselves. There was nothing more to talk about.

I tidied up things in the kitchen area, preparing the two remaining meds – morphine and decongestant – for the night ahead of me. Eventually, people started drifting off to their rooms. It was time to catch some sleep.

10 p.m. – I gave Karen a dose of morphine through her tube, set my alarm clock for midnight, and then climbed into the bed that Karen and I had shared for so many years. I got as close as I could to her, laying my hand on hers.

Midnight – my alarm clock rang. Time for morphine.

2 a.m. – alarm again. More morphine.

3 a.m. – I awoke to noise and movement. Karen was shifting around in her bed, agitated, restless, and uncomfortable. I did not get up right away, hoping that this was just a passing incident and that she would fall back asleep.

The opposite happened. Suddenly, she sat straight up in bed and continued the forward movement, hunched over, simultaneously breathing very hard and deep, as though suffocating.

Her deep inhales and exhales stunned me.

She was beside herself. A mess.

I bounded out of bed, alarm bells going off in my mind.

Apparently the morphine dose I had given Karen only an hour ago was no longer keeping her sedated, and now somewhat awake, she was literally fighting for every breath, fighting for her very life.

Yama looked at me, his eyes filled with the question: What is going on?

I texted Camile.

She responded immediately, "I am on my way."

Like a madman, I ran around the house, waking everyone up.

Someone called Neil.

And Ryan.

Karen was entering the last hours of her life.

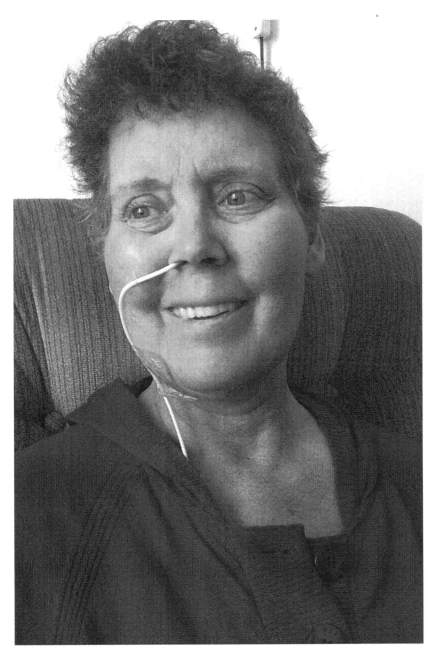

March 8, 2014 – Sandy home

~37~

Her Soul Departs

As Karen's race towards eternity accelerated, none of her family could have fully prepared themselves for the next six hours. Yet, as surely as the clock ticks, those terrible events were coming. It was an over-the-top intense, anguishing nightmare.

The specific details of Karen's last few hours on earth, starting early on the morning of March 11, began this book. Now, let me simply say that Karen's impending death – as daughter, wife, and mother – was likely the hardest test any of us had ever faced in our lives to date. At the same time, whether we knew it or not, accepted it or not, everyone there had already been granted supernatural strength and grace to deal with what is not normal, the passing of someone "before their time." I am absolutely convinced there is no other way we could have coped with what was before us.

After Camile and Neil's arrivals and Ryan's appearance via cyberspace, events cascaded from one unknown to another. There was no script. Karen's body and spirit, and her Creator were deciding what would happen next.

*****

9:15 a.m.

After a period of relative calm, Karen began sighing, deep, extended ones.

Allene and Amber, laying on the master bed just to Karen's right, drew close to their mother's body, as did Neil sitting in a chair on her left side, next to me. I was less than a foot away from her face, whispering in her ear, caressing her head, and occasionally kissing her. Through it all, her eyes remained wide open, unmoving, unblinking, focused upwards towards the ceiling.

A laptop computer sitting on a stool just to my right allowed Ryan to see his mother's face and hear everything as he joined us from Alaska, 5:15 a.m. local time.

Marjorie sat in a chair at her daughter's feet.

Over the next couple minutes, the sighing slowed.

We watched.

Waited.

Each person engrossed in a blizzard of thoughts and emotions.

As the seconds ticked by, it seemed she was pulling away, leaving us.

I whispered in her ear, "We love you, Karen. I love you. I will see you again soon."

One sigh was particularly deep.

She stilled.

Seconds later, another deep, reflexive sigh.

She stilled again.

Silence.

It was over.

At 9:30 a.m., a beautiful soul left us, gone to a Heavenly place, her new home.

Karen Allene Swan, age 56, who maintained a lifelong confidence that, at death, she would immediately go to be with her Savior, Jesus Christ, was now with Him.

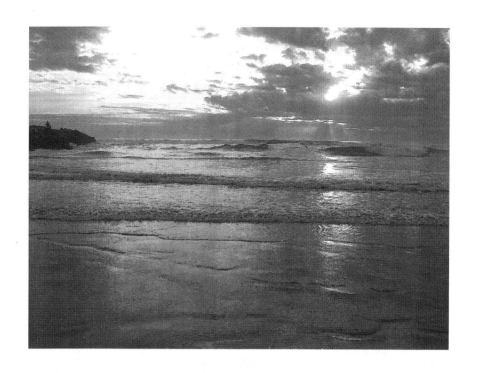

~38~

A Week of Preparations

9:31 a.m.

Ryan   Allene   Amber   Neil   Sterling   Marjorie

The six of us had just witnessed the death of a deeply beloved person – our wife, mother and daughter – and our lives would never been the same. In very personal, subconscious, even spiritual ways, we had changed.

What did this mean for us going forward? How would we grieve, this day, this week, at the funeral, and in the months ahead?

Who knew? Today is all we had, and on this day, events started moving at a rapid pace.

The first was Marjorie's imminent departure, plans made weeks ago when she agreed to fly up to help out. Who could have known how events would play out this past week?

When it became clear to me a couple of days ago that Karen could die any day, I asked Marjorie to stay longer. For reasons known only to her, she told me she wanted to return home as planned, to leave this very morning. Minutes after Karen died, I asked her again to stay, stating that I would buy her a new ticket. She said no. With that, my three children and I said our goodbyes, and by 10 a.m., she was gone, via a neighbor who the night before had agreed to run her to the airport.

I texted a few people, saying only, "Karen died today, at 9:30 a.m., at home." Within minutes, my cell phone was pinging like crazy with incoming texts. 45 arrived within the first hour alone. Among them was one from Bev Airhart, who was standing by at the Long Beach, California airport for my decision on whether she should fly up that day. That overlap – Marjorie going home, Bev coming – was planned before Karen's rapid decline the past weekend.

Now, overtaken by events, my head was spinning. What to do?

I told Bev to come, especially to comfort my daughters, help with the food preparations, and act as a sounding board as I planned the details for Karen's funeral.

As I made a couple urgent phone calls, Camile and my daughters removed Karen's feeding and catheter tubes, lightly bathed her, and slipped fresh clothes on her body. Camile then joined me in the kitchen, where we collected all Karen's liquid prescriptions, including some controlled substances, poured them all into a small plastic bag, and finally, added dish soap, neutralizing everything. For months those chemicals help keep her alive; now they were in a bag, worthless.

There was a metaphor in that. Our lives are equally frail and short, here today, gone tomorrow.

Lastly, she gave me details on when I could expect hospice staff to pick up the durable medical equipment – bed and infusion pump – and a few recommendations on managing the immediate grief, including an exhortation, "Get some sleep, Sterling."

Following hugs all around, Camile was gone.

Her job was over.

Utah law allows a deceased person's body to stay in a home for up to 24 hours. Morbid? On the contrary, it took a lot of pressure off me to quickly have Karen's body removed. Frankly, I was in no rush to move her. Some of my children wanted to sit with their mother's body.

Quietly.

In private.

That was completely understandable. I wanted the same and did, early in the afternoon.

Next, I called the mortuary. "Karen Swan has just died." Staff would come to my home that afternoon.

In the meantime, several courageous people came by to view Karen's body for the last time. I let each in, first to the living room, where they expressed their love to us, and then I walked each person into the master bedroom. Once there, I left each alone.

Jeff Nellermoe was out of town the coming weekend, so he and I settled on a Memorial Service date: Tuesday, March 18, at a local Sandy church.

Funeral preparations began. Ryan was flying in the next day. I implemented most of the suggestions Jeff had made regarding the funeral, ones we discussed during the weeks we had spent talking outside the house while Karen was still alive. His wisdom also helped me understand the needs and expectations of my four adult children. For a variety of reasons, these expectations posed some potential conflicts within my family, conflicts that required lots of patience and flexibility on the part of everyone.

Myself included.

Bev flew in that afternoon. Shortly after she got settled in at the house, two staff members from the mortuary knocked at my front door. They were polite, professional, and dressed in black. After signing the paperwork, they went out to their black Suburban, brought a four-wheeled gurney cart into my home and wheeled it into the master bedroom.

She still lay on the hospital bed. In clean clothes. Beautiful. At peace. One man carefully lifted her while another placed a tightly woven pad under her body. Then, with one man on each side of her, they carefully, respectfully, lifted her body off the hospital bed and to the gurney. A few steps later, Karen's body – not Karen Allene Swan, as she was somewhere else, completely healed – was placed in their Suburban, and with that, they left.

*****

Wednesday – I slept most of the day, occasionally getting up to enjoy the food that Bev made and touch base with my children. I was a physical and emotional mess. Allene, Amber, Ryan, and Neil were with friends, in different locales throughout the Salt Lake Valley.

Thursday – I had arranged for a final viewing of Karen's body, in one of her favorite dresses (selected by my daughters), which the staff placed on her, along with several favorite pieces of her jewelry, in a private room at the mortuary, located very close to my home. I instructed the funeral director not to do any embalming or cosmetic touch up.

Amber, Allene, and I rode to the Larkin mortuary on our bicycles, winding our way five miles around the Dimple Dell Wilderness Area, one of Karen's favorite recreation areas. We later agreed that Karen seemed to be riding with us. She would have loved that; it was just her style. My sons met us there.

"Where can we park our bikes," I asked the mortuary staff?

"What are you here for?"

"We have a private viewing scheduled for my wife," I answered.

They looked stunned. Mourners on bicycles? Dressed in bright bike clothes? The five Swans might have been sad, but were not giving up the things we loved.

We went into the viewing room, first as a family, and then each of us, alone, for about 15 minutes. Finally, we had invited two couples to come and view Karen, some of Karen's closest Utah friends.

Once the viewing ended, the five of us met at a local park for a family picture. If a picture is worth a thousand words, there are at least 5,000 words on the faces of my children and I in the picture taken that afternoon. We needed each other, and our grief was running deep.

Finally, we gathered in the living room at home, the place where we had spent so many years together as a family of six. On this afternoon, the topic was content and tone of Karen's memorial. For days, I had dreaded this necessary meeting, as expectations were all over the map, and I just didn't want things to boil over and explode. Suffice it to say that we had a respectful, spirited discussion about memorial issues large and small, such as types of music, who in the family would speak, what Jeff's short message would entail, service length, and when to show the video.

I listened, took a few notes, and then explained that the memorial would be overtly Christian, as this was Karen's core belief, the theme that she desired, made clear to me before she died. So it would be.

Planning complete, we parted ways for the evening.

It helped that everyone trusted Pastor Jeff Nellermoe. Over the next few days, he and I worked closely together via email on the myriad of memorial details (as he was out-of-town), weaving together a personal and spiritual funeral focus:

- Music
- Pastoral perspective
- Personal reflections
- A video highlighting Karen's married and maternal life
- And a light meal afterwards for all who attended.

As things took shape, I kept my children in the loop, and each helped make it happen, as they were able.

Friday - Karen's cremation was set for late morning. One moment I had wanted to drive to the crematorium to witness the process; the next minute, I wanted to avoid the place entirely. I had told the mortuary that we wanted Karen's ashes in two simple urns; an hour later, I called the coordinator and said one urn.

I was just beside myself; completely exhausted in every way. Fortunately, Ryan seized the initiative, drove to the mortuary's cremation facility, and observed some of the steps. We settled on two urns. That would prove wise once we finalized plans for spreading Karen's ashes.

I don't know what my other children did the rest of the day, but I slept.

*****

Saturday - Bev flew home in the morning. I slept off and on through the day.

Neil dropped by the house late Saturday morning, found me half awake in my bed, and asked if he could come in and "hang out" with me.

"Of course," I said. "Thank you."

It was a timely visit. By the weekend, communication between some of my children and I had reached a very raw point, so much so that I was probably depressed, something Neil picked up on.

Neil simply said, "You tried hard, Dad. Since I lived here, I saw what you did with Mom, more than anyone else. You did a good job."

His few comments, at age twenty-one, were precisely what I needed. They brought some peace to my very troubled soul.

Gail Kopetz, close family friend and gifted musician, one of the women who had flown out to spend time with Karen in January, flew in on Sunday. Amber's violin teacher picked her up from the airport, as together they would play a classical piece at the start of Karen's memorial.

Otherwise, plans continued to take shape for the memorial, including selecting pictures for a fifteen-minute video that we would show at the end of the service. Neil volunteered to pull everything together on his MacBook, and even in the midst of grieving for his mother, created an amazing record of Karen's life, principally her 7½-year cancer journey, that continues to inspire people to this day.

Dozens and dozens of calls, texts, cards, and even visits, poured in to the home from people expressing their sympathies. News spread via social media on the day and time of the memorial. Most impressive, Karen's sister, Rose, her husband, Bill, all their grown children, and one of Karen's other sister's daughters, spontaneously decided to converge on Sandy from Southern California. Many stayed in my home's basement beginning Sunday night. Their collective decision to all drop what they were doing and drive ten hours made a huge impression on my children and me.

These "travelers" lived out an important value: always, always try to "be there" for friends and family in need, even if they don't know how to ask for it. How we view ultimate reality, such as God, is often connected to how people love us when the chips are down. Frankly, I so wish more of Karen's immediate family would have attended the memorial. Theirs was a painful absence.

*****

On Monday, my children, friends and I pulled together the last few details for the music, speakers, pastoral role, video conclusion, and a post-service light meal at the church generously provided, free-of-charge for all guests, by Amber's former Great Harvest Bread owner/employer.

With that, the five Swans found ways to pass the time until the next morning, when we would be center stage in a memorial that was designed to honor a person we deeply loved, on one of the toughest days any of us had ever faced.

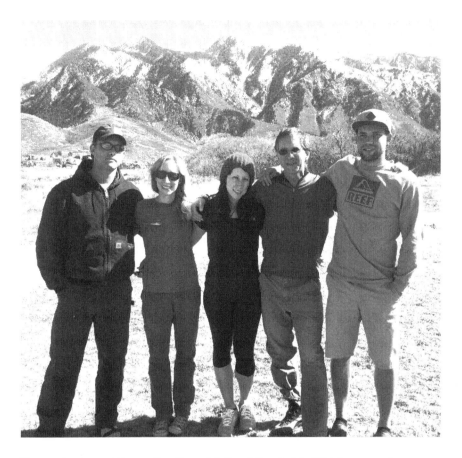

Ryan, Amber, Allene, Sterling, Neil – March 13, 2014 – two days after Karen's death

~39~

"Karen Will Always be in My Heart"

Tuesday, March 18, 2014, 10:30 a.m.

As extended family, long-time friends, former students, Karen's circle of fellow cancer survivors, neighbors, employers, several of my former FAA co-workers, and staff from the Huntsman Cancer Hospital converged on Sandy's Good Shepherd Lutheran Church for the memorial, my children and I gathered with Pastor Jeff Nellermoe in a small room off the main church lobby. Jeff reminded us of the order of service, drew us together as only a pastor could, even as we might have wanted to run away, and offered up a brief prayer.

A minute before 11 a.m., he led us into the church's sanctuary, filled, we later found out, with over 175 people of all ages, who had come to honor Karen and support the five of us. I looked neither left nor right as my children and I walked to the front of the sanctuary, where we sat, together, in a pew.

Jeff walked to the front platform, turned around to face the audience, and with that, the service began. First, Judy and Gail performed a beautiful violin/piano duet. Next came a short devotional talk by Pastor Nellermoe, using as his reference one of Karen's cross stitch crafts, on the theme of God's promises, art that had hung in our master bedroom for years.

Following this were short, very personal reflections about Karen by each of my four children, as well as her sister, Rose, and Karen's close friend, Gail. I did not speak because the memories were too raw.

Pastor Jeff returned for some final words, drawing everyone's attention to four verses from the Bible, a fitting way to accent Karen's faith in God's promises while inviting others to see them, too. Then, the lights dimmed and a 15-minute video, celebrating Karen's life, primarily as a married woman, ran on the sanctuary's large screens.

One of my nephews offered a short, heartfelt closing prayer, which ended the memorial service.

It was a few minutes before noon.

Guests remained in their seats as the five of us got up and headed towards the lobby of the church, Ryan in the lead. He let out a loud, raw wail as he briskly walked towards the lobby of the church, out the exterior doors, and kept on going. His wail expressed how I felt, too.

One of my neighbors, also Ryan's friend, went looking for him. My three other children headed for other parts of the church's large lobby or fellowship hall, as I stopped just outside the sanctuary doors, waiting for what was to come next.

While I stood there, and as Pastor Jeff invited the guests to gather for food in the fellowship hall, something completely unexpected occurred in a matter of just ten seconds.

A middle-aged man walked purposefully up to me from a corner of the lobby. He was a mystery person; I had never met him before. He shook my hand, offered his condolences, and said, "I was just at a funeral last week for a person from another religion, and it was all gloom and hopelessness, as speaker after speaker voiced worry about whether this deceased person had done enough good deeds to get into Heaven. Today's memorial, celebrating Karen's life, was hopeful and filled with the love of life. Thank you."

With that, he walked out the door and was gone. I never saw him again.

*****

Next thing I knew, friends, some I had not seen in years, lining up to express their condolences, shake my hand or give me a big hug. One after another, people came, patiently waited, and then, in their own ways, spoke glowingly of Karen while showering me with love. I stood in that lobby for what seemed an hour, deeply moved by those who cared enough to come that day. It was a mind-blowing time; words fall short.

At one point, Joan, Karen's favorite Huntsman Cancer Hospital nurse practitioner, came up to greet me. We talked quietly for a few moments, and then, during a sustained hug, she whispered in my ear, "Karen will always be in my heart." I knew this would be true.

Waiting behind Joan were Patrick and Kimberly, Karen's Huntsman Hospital Exercise Trainers, two amazing human beings who tapped into Karen's love of physical activity, assisting her in her statistics-busting fight with advanced stage melanoma.

*****

By 1 p.m., most of the guests were gone. Great Harvest had done a phenomenal job feeding everyone. After I grabbed some leftovers, my children and I loaded personal items into my car, and off we went, some to my home, some to their apartments, and others, to spend time with friends.

Karen's sister, Rose, and her extended family met me at my house. People settled in, relaxing after an intense morning, as Rose and others started cooking a meal for this small army. My daughters soon arrived, as did Gail, and later, most piled into cars and headed up Little Cottonwood Canyon, just to hang out and let off steam.

Later that evening, everyone gathered around my large dining room table for dinner. It was then that one of my neighbors dropped in and, with tears in her eyes, read the contents of a gift from Karen to my children and me. It was a small plaque, whose words expressed Karen's love for her family, her joy in her new Heavenly home, and hope that we move on in life.

It was a simple, powerful message. Tears flowed freely. They still do in me to this day when I read the words.

Dinner over and night falling, my house guests, now just the Zellmer family, went to various corners of my first and basement floors and occupied themselves, while I hid in my room. The shock of what happened the past seven days, especially that morning, finally had caught up with me.

I started to grieve.

Hard.

Overwhelmed, exhausted, and disoriented, I did not ask for help, even though Bill, my favorite brother-in-law, was in the house not 25 feet away. I stayed holed up in my room until it was time for bed.

Early the next morning, the Zellmers left for Southern California. Suddenly, the house was quiet. Only Allene was staying there. My adult children and I needed some space following the previous intense 24 hours, so we agreed to meet for dinner at a restaurant the next evening to discuss plans for scattering Karen's ashes. Other than going over to the mortuary to pick up the two urns, I have no recollection of what I did the next day and a half. My mind was blank, my heart, broken.

*****

Thursday night came; time to gather for dinner. Again, I was anxious. Even though everyone was respectful of one another in the lead-up to the memorial, during the service, and afterwards, I was feeling self-conscious because I had been indecisive when it came to some group arrangements these last few weeks, and some of my children had made it known that they were in no mood to have me change my mind once again when it came to the subject of their mom's ashes.

Dinner around that large table was part food, part brainstorming, and part agreeing on a plan and committing to making it work. The plan? Scatter the ashes in two places, Utah and California, half on Mother's Day, the other half on September 4, Karen's birthday. Ryan was uncertain whether he could attend the Mother's Day scattering, but along with the rest of us, committed to Oceanside in six months.

Clearly, anticipatory grief, where each of us had been a part of a seven-year journey caused by evil cancer, had reached a climax. Karen was dead. Going forward, each of us would grieve her absence in very personal ways.

Yet, life had to go on.

Karen wanted it so.

The next morning, Ryan left for Alaska, and Allene, Oregon. Amber, living in her own place 30 minutes away, went back to work. Neil returned to his university dorm. My home, the scene of so much intensity, especially recently, was now eerily quiet.

Six months later, the five of us would gather together again.

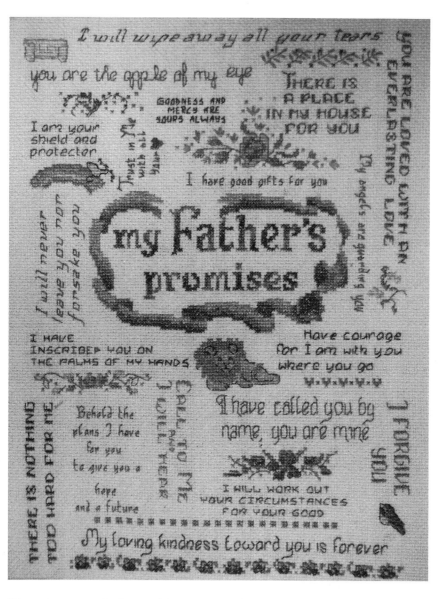

Karen's cross-stitch, used by Pastor Jeff in the Memorial Service

~40~

Scattering Her Ashes

<u>The Wilderness Area</u>

The Heavens were weeping on this Mother's Day Sunday morning in mid-May 2014. Last March, my children and I had agreed that Mother's Day was when we would spread half of Karen's ashes.

Spreading the ashes in the Wasatch mountains just east of my home was our first choice, but everything there was still snow packed, so we went with an alternate, the Dimple Dell Wilderness Area, a half mile from my home and one of Karen's favorite locations. She had spent hundreds of hours there, walking by herself, with family, the family dog, and riding horses with Allene, Amber or Mim Nellermoe. It was a fitting place to return part of her body.

A light rain had fallen all night, and as Allene, Amber, Neil and I walked through a trailhead gate into the Area, low hanging clouds from the lingering storm collided with each other and the mountains to create the sense, at least in me, that God himself was aware of us mourning our beloved wife and mother. The turbulent weather, wet soil, towering mountains, dormant foliage and absolute quiet provided a fitting setting as we walked to a high point on the trail and then agreed on how we would go about spreading the ashes.

I went first, carefully opening the plastic urn that had sat in my bedroom closet since last March. Then, with Neil's help, I removed the clear plastic bag that contained half of her cremains. My hands were shaking, and not from the cold.

Bag in hand, I walked alone down towards the stream-cut gully, below, and then stopped about 100' away from my three children. There, to my left, in a sandy berm, was a spring wildflower poking its head above the brown bushes. That became my chosen spot. As I carefully poured my ¼ ash amount, I talked out loud to Karen, to

God, to anyone who was listening. Once done, I stood still, quiet, lost in thought.

Eventually, I walked back up the hill to where my children were standing. Amber went next. She, too, walked down the hill, chose her resting spot for Karen's ashes, and after a short while returned.

Allene and Neil chose another spot in this expansive, open Area, each spreading the ashes, each reflecting in a very personal way.

Finally, the cremation bag was empty. Half of Karen's body had been left in the moist Wilderness Area soil. More rain later that afternoon would complete the process. Together we walked the short distance back to the car, which I had parked at the trailhead gate, and drove home.

Or at least tried! I was so lost in thought that I nearly missed a turn to the feeder street by my home, a road I had correctly turned on thousands of times over the last many years.

Truly, a heavy heart does strange things.

Sea Star, Oceanside, September 4

Although Karen was born in Grand Rapids, Michigan, her family moved to North County San Diego in the mid-1960s, at that time, a semi-rural area. She grew up with a deep love for the ocean, a love that stayed with her throughout her life.

It was this love that explains why the Sea Star fishing boat caught her eye following the melanoma diagnosis. The boat's home port was Oceanside harbor, 15 minutes from her folk's Vista home, and a banner near the dock said, "Burials At Sea." Early on, she decided that was what she wanted when she died.

So it would be.

*****

It had been nearly six months since my children and I had all been together, almost four since Amber, Allene, Neil and I scattered the first half of Karen's ashes in the Wilderness Area on Mother's Day morning. Much had happened during that short interlude: Allene was now living near Ventura/Santa Barbara, California; Amber had moved to Northern Virginia; Ryan was still in Alaska, but not for much longer; and Neil was still attending the University of Utah.

On Thursday afternoon, September 4 – Karen's 57th birthday – the five of us converged on Oceanside to spread Karen's ashes at sea. The weather was ideal, and the harbor, quiet, which provided a helpful counterpoint to the upheaval going on, to one degree or another, in each of our spirits. Although the boat could hold up to sixty passengers, for a variety of reasons, we only wanted the five of us on the water together, explaining early on to family and friends our preference.

We had gathered a handful of 8x10 pictures of Karen, colorful flowers, several bags of flower petals, and, at the captain's suggestion, I brought an iPod with some music. Several family members preferred silence, so we went with that. Good call.

Joe, the Sea Star's captain, ran two unrelated businesses off one boat, sport fishing trips out in the Pacific during the day, and evening burials at sea. The two "worlds" were not an obvious fit, but during a phone conversation with Joe early in the spring, I got a good read on his personality, education, 20 years of experience on the water, and awareness of grieving families' needs.

Within five minutes, I was convinced that Captain Joe was the right guy for our needs. This was a new, intense experience for Amber, Allene, Neil, Ryan and I, and this man, although apparently not a church pastor, would know how to help us navigate the many challenges my family would have as we headed out to open water.

As the clock struck 5 p.m., Joe met me at the dock where we discussed a few last-minute details. Then, he assisted Allene and Amber as they tastefully arranged the photos and flowers on the stern (rear of the boat), along with the urn containing the second half of Karen's cremains, as Ryan, Neil and I waited on shore.

*****

Finally, it was time. As we gathered on the stern, Joe introduced himself to the family and briefed us what we could expect, including:

- After exiting the harbor, he would take us directly west about three miles, kill the diesel engines, and let the boat drift
- Each of us would scatter a portion of the ashes
- After all the ashes were scattered, we would continue to drift for a few more minutes

- Next, he would start the engines, circle the drifting ashes and flowers as they were carried by the tide
- Finally, we would head back to land.

As the powerful diesel engines kicked in and the boat slowly made its way into the harbor channel, the five of us gathered at various spots along the perimeter of the Sea Star's deck. There was lots of harbor activity as we slowly headed out beyond the breakwater, but my mind was a million miles away. Suddenly, I was pulled back to the present. Two ocean-going outrigger canoe teams began shadowing the Sea Star for a short ways, and then fell behind as we accelerated. For a moment, I thought I saw Karen in one of those giant canoes.

Soon, we were in open, calm water. The sun, slowly setting to the west, was still bright and warming. Out in the vast Pacific, away from "civilization," the senses became saturated, allowing each of us to drift into our own realms. Occasionally, my children and I would exchange a few words, hugs, or simply stand next to one another. Overall, the engine's roar, waves hitting the bow as we headed into open water, and the plaintive cry of gulls, was enough. Captain Joe and his deckhand remained in the wheelhouse as we headed out, providing us the privacy we sought.

At one point Ryan and I wound up standing next to each other. Looking out on the water as he spoke, he precisely captured the place and mood, saying, "This is exactly where we should be, Dad" (spoken with a bit more colorful language). I wholeheartedly agreed.

About three miles out, nearly directly west of Oceanside's pier, Captain Joe killed the engines, their roar suddenly replaced with intense sounds of silence. As I looked east towards the coast, where everything looked small, toy-like, memories flooded back to the many days Karen and the kids had spent playing on that idyllic beach. Just about a year ago, she and I had walked together to the very end of the pier.

The Sea Star drifted, bobbing lightly with the waves. I looked around. We were nearly alone.

Captain Joe joined us on the stern as we gathered around a small, 5'x5' raised area on which laid pictures of Karen, flowers, and the urn. He asked if I wanted to make any remarks. I did not.

No words could capture my thoughts at that moment, much less any ability I might have to express anything relevant to my four adult children. He stepped into that vacuum. Based on years of experience, he made a few brief observations that stay with me to this day. In summary, he said:

- Look at that coastline three miles to the east of us. Forty years ago, there was almost nothing there; now look at the significant human development. Out on the water, there is no human development. This is nature in its raw form.
- San Diego County has millions of people. Out here, on the water, there is our boat, and in the distance, two small sailboats. That's it, for far as our eyes can see.
- The Pacific Ocean's waters connect with all the other oceans of the world, so that wherever you are in the world, if you have access to an ocean, Karen's cremains are symbolically there, too.

With that, he gave us instructions. He would stand at a corner of the stern, holding the plastic bag containing Karen's ashes. One by one, each family member would move up next to him, and together, the two would take the bag, lean over the railing, and slowly drop about ⅕ of the ash into the water. While this was happening, other family members could drop flowers and Rose petals into the water, since these would float along with the ash, creating a powerful effect.

"Who would like to go first?"

I can't remember the sequence, only that I wanted to go last.

It was time. The simple, solemn ceremony began. As the ash dropped into the water, the ocean's invisible current carried those small, gray particles to the left of our boat, out to sea, as it also did the flowers and petals. Currents of tears flowed down our faces.

As one of my children finished, another stepped forward.

Soon, the combination of ash and flowers created a narrow, serpentine trail towards open water. For some reason, the ash turned nearly fluorescent as it hit the water.

Stunning.

Finally, it was my turn. To my right was Captain Joe, with the bag, contents almost gone. We bent over the railing together, our four hands firmly clasping the open bag.

My hands shook.

Tears flowed, covering my glasses, making it somewhat difficult for me to see.

Slowly, deliberately, I poured out the remaining ash.

Eventually, the bag flapped in the breeze.

It was empty.

Captain Joe headed back to the wheelhouse, started up the diesel engines, and then ever so slowly encircled the daisy-chain of glowing ash and multi-colored flowers, the ash just inches below the water's surface, the flowers, floating obediently along on top. By now this chain was over 100 feet long, Karen's ashes heading out into the deep ocean that she so loved so much.

Our formal goodbye to Karen over, it was time to head back to the harbor. Captain Joe pointed the boat towards shore, and as we accelerated, once again the ocean dosed us with spray. At one point, I stood on the stern watching the ash daisy chain fade from view, and suddenly broke into uncontrollable hard crying.

Ryan walked over, wrapped his arm around me and kept it there for a long time. I still feel that arm.

As we drew close to the harbor, part of me was hoping that something dramatic, even supernatural, might happen, like the morning Jeff and Mim Nellermoe were directed to enter our home the day Karen died. As the Sea Star drew closer and closer to the harbor, my hope started to fade.

Suddenly, out of nowhere, a large pod of dolphins joined our little boat as it sped towards land, darting all around us, especially near the bow (front), for what seemed several minutes. These magnificent mammals were some of Karen's favorites, and here they were, escorting us, and yes, even bringing some joy, after a very heavy time just a few minutes earlier.

"His voice is on the waters…" says a verse in the Book of Psalms, Old Testament. So it was, for me at least, via his representatives, dolphins.

*****

Once docked, the five of us ate dinner at Rockin' Baja, one of Karen's favorite restaurants on the Oceanside Harbor. It was a bittersweet time, the final minutes of a memorial day for a woman we dearly loved. At the table, we exchanged small talk. It was enough. One final memory drew the day to a close; a brilliant sunset filled the sky just as we finished our meals.

So fitting.

As the red and orange hues turned to gray, we parted ways; Ryan heading off to spend a few hours with a cousin in the area, while the rest of us went back to my in-laws' home. After some small talk with them, Allene, Amber, Neil and I headed off to bed, as tomorrow the five of us would part ways once again.

Next morning Amber, Neil and I were up early, driving north along the coast, heading first to John Wayne airport, Amber's departure point back to Northern Virginia. After dropping her off, Neil and I kept going, to Long Beach airport, where I ditched the rental car and we flew home to Salt Lake City. Allene and Ryan drove to Allene's home in Santa Paula, near Ventura, to spend a few days together.

We had reached closure.

Sort of.

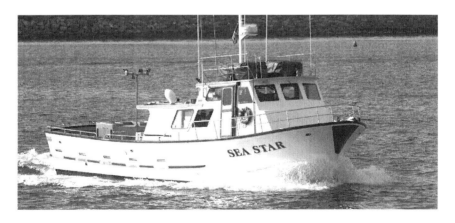

Oceanside Harbor, CA

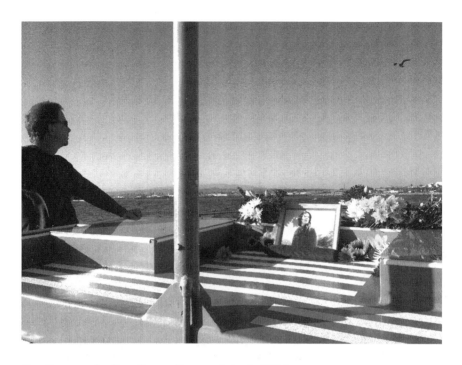

Sterling on the Sea Star – September 4, 2014

~41~

Life After Death…

An ER physician's comment, "That should not be there," started this whole horrible cancer journey way back in the fall of 2006. These five words suddenly blew Karen, Allene, Amber, Ryan, Neil and I onto the road less traveled, where our lives, individually and collectively, would change in ways that we could scarcely imagine.

Similarly, when the clock struck 9:30 a.m. on March 11, 2014, another strong gust of wind at once lifted Karen up into the loving arms of her Creator, while leaving my children and I on earth. What did it mean to grieve and hope, to process all the memories and feelings of nearly eight long years, while coming to terms with what we thought about life and God, that is, if we thought there was a God at all?

Psychologists often talk about stages of grief – denial, anger, bargaining, depression, and acceptance – and emphasize that the first year of a loss is often the most difficult, since life's normal milestones and celebrations, such as birthdays, holidays, and anniversaries, add to the already intense memories and sense of loss. In my experience, these grief "stages" are not linear; I find myself in one stage, then like a whiplash, flip back to an earlier one.

What about the second year? How was that? I recall it a little less intense, but no less painful. In fact, the ache I felt in Year 2 following Karen's death was actually deeper, albeit less frequent. While I cried less, when I did, it's like someone had punched me in the chest.

Since part of grieving is remembering, it was fitting that Amber and Allene flew to Utah the first weekend in June 2015 for a Little Red Riding Hood memorial ride, this time choosing the 75-mile route option. I tagged along, volunteering with other men to make the Ride run smoothly for the 3,500 female participants. There they were, my beautiful twin daughters, riding strong together, honoring their mom.

*****

This year, Year 3, has brought times of surprising joy and laughter to my life, but I still find myself randomly thinking, "I can't believe she is gone," often spoken out loud, very loud, when no one else is around. Sometimes I yell it at God. So it goes.

I cannot speak for my children, how each of them is coping as the distance grows, day by day, from that fateful March morning, but I see some encouraging trends, for at least three reasons:

First, my children and I, although separated by physical distance, are working at staying in touch with each other. Social media, texting, frequent phone calls, and occasional face-to-face visits make it convenient; desire makes it happen.

Second, I believe spreading Karen's ashes off the California coast in 2014 started the process of repairing relationships that became strained during her long illness, especially during the final couple years. This "warming trend" continues. We are trying to forgive, affirm, and even occasionally laugh. These are all good things.

Third, Colleen, my wise, widowed younger sister, told me right after Karen died, "Ster, I have two pieces of advice: 1) The most you can do for your children is pray for them; 2) You must focus on making changes in your own life – hope, joy, faith, purpose, giving. As you do, your children will see it. Do not preach. Actions speak louder than words."

After Karen died, I did not want to hear either one of those two suggestions. Her long cancer journey was like someone throwing a hand grenade in the midst of my family, disorienting everyone. After she was finally gone, I so wanted everything to get back to "normal," whatever that was.

That was foolish thinking. Colleen was right. After over two years, I affirm that things take time. I now understand that in my human experience, it is mostly about time, but in God's plan, it is all about timing. He often takes longer than I would prefer, yet when he does move, it's dramatic.

*****

Currently, my children are living all over the United States:

- Amber lives in Northern Virginia, working full-time as a pastry chef at a cool restaurant that distributes her handiwork to many other sales outlets. Among other things, she enjoys riding on many of the area's renowned bike paths.
- Allene lives in Santa Paula, California, earning her living as a respected dog groomer at a large animal hospital, and loves the easy access to the ocean.
- Ryan lives in Maui, Hawaii, working as an airframe and powerplant technician maintaining helicopters, requiring impressive skills and high ethical standards. In his off hours, he explores the island by bicycle, motorcycle, and foot.
- Neil continues his civil engineering education at the University of Utah. Newly married, this exciting event brought my family back together again for the first time in nearly two years. It was a time of great celebration and joy.

I worked at Alta Ski Area's Ticket Office this past ski season, fielding phone calls from customers all over the country. It was a blast, a low-stress job filled with lots of laughter in a beautiful setting.

Fortunately, I have several new irons in the job fire, opportunities that dovetail with my personality, interests, life experience, and convictions about what really matters in life. On most days, I enjoy life. Karen is my example. When I tell her story, people are moved in a powerful way, to love, to hope, to make choices that have eternal significance.

*****

Karen, a determined Dutch woman who pushed back against cancer, engaged in life, loved her husband, children, and others, while maintaining faith in Christ that both convicted and inspired me, is the reason this book is written. It is my attempt at an unvarnished, straightforward, generous record of her incredible journey against all odds.

The words came in bursts to me over these past two years. Sometimes I would write like a man possessed. Other times I took weeks, even months off, usually grieving heavily during those lull times, or even getting directly in God's face and arguing about the wisdom of taking my wife before her time.

Oh, well. Some things are not for me to decide.

For those that knew Karen, loved her, served her, or perhaps are learning about her for the first time, thank you for reading this book about the best human relationship I ever had. She was a good one, a keeper. The singer, Joni Mitchell, says it best, "Don't it always seem to go that you don't know what you've got 'til it's gone."

I wrote this book largely to honor Karen Allene Swan and document her journey for my children. Secondarily, I wrote it to testify about a God who cares, who loves us in the midst of our human experience, who carried the Swans along during those long, turbulent, horrible, joyous, life-shaping years.

Perhaps you don't believe in God or are alienated from him. I can't speak for your journey. All I know is that the events these years cannot merely be explained through reason, coincidence, fate, karma, serendipity, clever timing, or some quid pro quo with a distant Being. Something else was going on, beyond just the Swan family, friends, extraordinary medical care or Nature, and I felt it necessary to speak honestly about this.

The fact is each of our lives is short, like a vapor. What, really, is the purpose of life? In my view, it is certainly more than just putting in time, accumulating things, or completing a Bucket List.

Karen gave me 33 memorable years of marriage and four priceless children, and if I can trust Jesus's words, I will see her again.

She was the woman in the bed.

Knowing, serving and loving her changed my life.

"For God so loved the world, that he gave his only son, that whoever believes in him will not perish, but have everlasting life." Jesus's words - from the Gospel of John, The Bible.

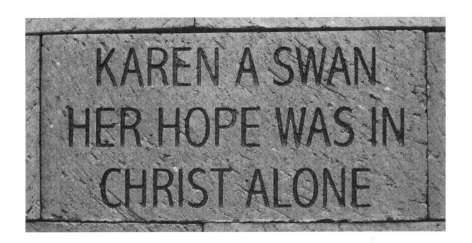

Paver stone placed in Karen's honor – in an alcove at the Huntsman Cancer Hospital.

Appendix:
Who was Karen Swan?

She was born Karen Allene Scheltema, in Grand Rapids, Michigan, on September 4, 1957, the first of four children, three girls, one boy. Her parents took Karen and her two younger sisters to British Guyana in the early 60's, where they served as missionaries for a year. After that experience, they returned to the United States and eventually relocated to North County San Diego, California, where Karen grew up.

As a Southern California girl, Karen had lots of opportunities for outside exploration, and she made the most of it. She developed a love of nature, animals, horseback riding, the ocean, and other cultures, especially anything with a Latin influence. In addition, Karen grew to love music – learning to play both the piano and violin – and excelled in many high school sports. Intensely curious, she also did well academically, deciding to attend Biola University in La Mirada, CA, majoring in Liberal Studies so she could go into elementary education.

Raised in a Christian home, Karen had her eye on teaching overseas in a missionary children's (MK) school, when she met her future husband, Sterling Swan, in the summer of 1979 when they were on the same team during a summer missions program in Central America. Married a year later, Sterling and Karen's church sent them to India in 1981 for nine months. Lots of other international travel followed, but India would be a life-shaping event in their lives.

After returning to the United States, Sterling started a career with the Federal government, which required them to move to Salt Lake City, Utah, where they would spend most of the next thirty years. There, she had four children, two boys, and twin girls, pouring her life into their lives, the community, local churches, homeschool co-ops, music lessons for her children, and of course, lots and lots of outdoor activities that would shape her children's lives. In addition, Karen was extremely creative, in cooking, sewing, and arts of all kinds, something evident in every corner of her home, and again, in the lives of her children.

She taught her children by doing things with them. Some of the best years were on Utah's renown snow-covered slopes right up the canyon from her home. During the winters, Ryan, Amber, Allene and Neil learning how to ski, snowboard and snowshoe. During the summers, it was all about exploration in the mountains, or bicycle riding, hiking local trails, going camping, or visiting national parks. Her Sandy home became a creative spot, still true to this day. Just drive by her home, look at the front yard, and on display is Karen's personality.

At Karen's core were a zest for life, a deep curiosity about everything, optimistic outlook on life and challenges, and an abiding love for God and His promises of life with Him – now and after death. Even after her Stage IV melanoma cancer diagnosis in October 2006, she would not go quietly into the night. Her determination to live, for her children and husband, assisted by the prayers of many, plus the expertise of staff at the Huntsman Cancer Hospital, meant that she survived this deadly disease long after the statistics said she should have died.

Karen passed away at home on March 11, 2014. She was a woman who loved her God, her husband, children and friends, and life itself.

Extend Her Legacy?

Would you like to support cancer research in Karen's memory?

When giving to the Huntsman Cancer Foundation, 100% of your contribution goes to cancer research at the Huntsman Cancer Institute.

To donate, go to the Huntsman Cancer Institute web site:

www.huntsmancancer.org

Thank you.

*****

About the author:

Sterling Swan was born and raised in Southern California. In the mid-1970's, he moved to the San Fernando Valley, CA for further education. Among other things, he met Karen Scheltema in Central America on a Practical Missionary Training team in the summer of 1979. They fell in love and married a year later.

Sterling has two younger sisters, four grown children, and currently lives in Salt Lake City, Utah. He enjoys the outdoors, bicycling, and humor.

This is his first book.

Made in the USA
Lexington, KY
11 January 2017